Baby's First-Year Milestones

How To Take Care of Your Baby Effectively, Track Their Monthly Progress And Ensure Their Physical, Mental And Brain Development Are on The Right Track

By

Harley Carr

Having a child is one of life's great joys. As you watch your baby grow you will be amazed by not only their physical development but also their emotional development. So much growth happens on both levels as your child is in what is considered the "first-year" of life. Baby's first year is a year of wonder and firsts. First smile, first word, first solid food, first tentative steps, and many more—as your baby explores their environment and learns about the world. It's important to document your baby's milestones, not only to capture their magical moments but also for medical reasons.

Track your little one's milestones with this free **"Baby's Milestones Journal".**

With everything the baby does for the first time, it can be difficult to decide which events are worth recording. It's also easy to miss an important baby's milestones in the chaos of new parenthood. So we've compiled a list of suggestions on how to document baby's first year and which milestones are worth documenting.

Get your **"Baby's Milestones Journal"** in PDF format by clicking the link below:

https://harleycarrparenting.com/babys-first-year-milestones/

or

Print the document and start to record your baby's important milestones and events.

This printable Baby's Milestones Journal is available in both "Baby Girl" and "Baby Boy" version.

Now, you can have your *easy to fill in* "Baby's Milestones Journal " in just one click away!

Let´s get started ...

Enjoy and Best Wishes to your parenting journey!

Harley Carr

Table of Contents

Introduction

Expecting a newborn is simultaneously one of the most exciting, yet most terrifying, moments of life as parents. Get ready! Your life is about to change in all the best ways. After the pregnancy is over and the delivery has happened, you are then catapulted into the role of being a parent to this being that is brand new to the world. From here, you need to teach this baby everything that they need in order to become a successful adult. A lot of expecting parents feel that they do not have enough information in order to feel confident in their abilities as parents – this is a problem. With all that you can discover through reading this guide, you will be more prepared than ever when it comes to welcoming your newborn into your life. Instead of questioning your ability to raise a baby, you will be excited and happy to teach your little one everything there is to know about the world.

After the delivery, it will feel as time is going to speed up. After being pregnant for so many months, holding your baby in your arms for the first time is a surreal experience. You might have to turn to your partner in disbelief at the fact that you two were responsible for the joy that is now your newborn. Your baby will be measured and cleaned, and any additional testing or aftercare will be performed. A short stay in the hospital will likely occur, and then you are sent home to begin life as parents. Not only do you have to get used to being a caretaker, but your baby is also getting used to a new environment. After spending so many months inside the womb, you can imagine how foreign everything looks and feels to the baby as they are brought into their home for the first time.

You will go through many sleepless nights, listen to crying that can't seem to be soothed by any solution that you can think of, and panic at the thought that you are doing something wrong. These are all normal aspects of parenthood, and you shouldn't feel ashamed or guilty if you go through any of these things. Though you won't always have all of the answers, you will figure out the solutions as you go. Guides like this one exist so that you can take the guesswork out of parenting. Instead of feeling clueless and helpless, you will be able to use your knowledge as power in order to take care of your new baby. The information that you receive will act as the foundation for how you wish to shape your child.

A lot of what you hear about doing the "right" thing for your baby is going to come from other people in your life or what society views as the "norm." While these opinions and the advice given to you might be helpful, it can also be hindering and confusing. Instead of letting other people tell you how to take care of your child, you can inform yourself in order to make the best decisions possible on your own terms. This is a confidence boost in itself! You will be able to navigate parenting with ease, and not to mention, you will also have fun while doing so. At the end of the day, parenting should be taken in a lighthearted manner. Enjoy all of the milestones and learn from the mistakes that are made – no one is a perfect parent, but an involved parent will raise a wonderful child.

You cannot redo the first year of your baby's life. This is the groundwork that you are responsible for putting down in order for your baby to grow up to be a thriving and independent child. It is a lot of pressure to think about the bigger picture, but don't let this scare you. With the knowledge that you have already, plus the knowledge that you will gain from reading this book, you will be able to approach parenting with ease by being able to have faith in yourself. You should *know* that your decisions are the right decisions.

Practical Solutions

This guide is meant to teach you everything that you really need to know about being a great parent. There are no gimmicks or promises with no proof to back them up; all you will find here are real tips and methods that are meant to make your life easier and your baby happier and healthier. As you learn this useful information, you will be taught exactly how to take care of your child as soon as the delivery takes place. This is a time when most parents are filled with a rush of adrenaline. Everyone is going to want to meet your new baby, and it will be a joy to show them off. You will be filled with happiness because of all the excitement. Once this socialization period has ended and you are left alone to care for your baby for the very first time, this can admittedly be a scary time for a lot of people. Thus begins the feeling of wondering, "What do I do now?"

A lot of parents agree that the nurse placing your baby in your arms for the first time is both overwhelmingly emotional and utterly terrifying. Many mothers, at this moment, realize that they are now responsible for the life that they are holding. While your baby grew and developed inside of your stomach for all of those months, you had little control over what happened. While you took care of yourself and ate a proper diet, your baby did the rest. Now, the tables have turned. It is your chance to lead your baby toward the best developmental decisions. You can show your baby what to do and how to behave in this world.

As your baby grows, you will be guided through what you must know in order to effortlessly get them through their first year of life. From what vaccines and vitamins are essential to whether or not you should opt for diagnostic testing, these topics will be discussed in detail for you to make your own decisions. By taking this initiative, you are already being a great parent. You will also learn about the essentials, such as how to buy the right diapers, clothing, equipment, and more. It makes sense to start from the beginning because your baby will also be starting from the very beginning. You will be learning together, every step of the way.

One of the best things that you will learn by reading this guide is how to differentiate truths from myths during your baby's first year. There is a lot of information circulating around that pertains to what a child *should* be able to do at certain points in life. By actually realizing that each child is going to develop differently and that it is normal, it will help to put you at ease as you compare your baby's progress to that of the average child. A unique path of development means that milestones are going to be reached when the time is right. Know that your baby is born with certain instincts, so they also know what they are doing.

Learning what is true and important will keep you on track and, in turn, make you a better parent. Instead of getting stuck on the what-ifs, you will be able to recognize that childhood can be unpredictable. All you can do is your best, and that is how to be the best for your child. Remember that you and your partner are responsible for making the decisions. No matter what you read or what you hear, you both know your baby best. Starting from day one, you will learn about all of their habits and quirks. It will likely be impossible to put the camera down as you attempt to capture each of these nuances.

There is no such thing as a guide that contains all of the answers, this one included. Parenting has a lot to do with discovery, and this is something that you will need to do on your own. After reading this guide, you will have the essential tools that you can use to guide you in the right direction. You need to show your baby that you know what you are doing, even though you might be thinking that you actually don't — fake it till you make it! With these solutions, you will be less likely to make as many mistakes. Though mistakes are an important learning experience, you don't need to make hundreds of them in order to be considered an experienced parent.

My Story

I am Harley Carr, a proud mother of three. I have been a parent for 8 years now, starting with the birth of my son. He changed my entire life, an unexpected blessing at a time that I didn't exactly have a plan. Years later, I had more children. Though they were in my plan this time, they each made me a better mother in their own ways. My 5-year old and 3-year old do their best to keep me in check, teaching me new things every single day. Having many children can be difficult, especially with these age gaps, but being their mother is something that I truly enjoy. I can say, without a doubt, that being their mother is my greatest accomplishment in life thus far. My journey has not been all sunshine and rainbows. As a mother, I faced quite a few difficulties.

During the first year of each child's life, so many decisions needed to be made. Nobody warns you of exactly how many decisions you will have to make during this year. Will you bottle feed or breastfeed? Do you plan on practicing attachment parenting? Are you going to secure childcare after your maternity leave is over? One of the hardest decisions that I personally had to make was when to return to my job. I loved my job, but through giving birth to my first son, I realized that I wanted to give him all that I could. I ended up leaving my position as a psychologist and becoming a full-time mom instead. I stayed at home with him each day, getting to know him better than I ever thought I'd be able to.

My days went from sitting at a desk to sitting in a rocking chair. I held my baby, soothed my baby, and fed my baby at all hours of the day. I was able to regulate a schedule that we could both follow, making it easier for us to eat and sleep together. This was the majority of what happened in the first year of motherhood. I enjoyed this so much, and I was thankful that I had a partner who was willing to support me as I stayed at home with our newborn son. The memories that we made at home together were some that I will never forget.

For each of my children, I truly saw the value of breastfeeding. They were all breastfed, and as they began to grow up, I could see the benefits. All 3 of my children have been generally healthy with strong immune systems. It has been quite a journey, raising these three children, and I could not have done it without the help of my dedicated partner. In this guide, I hope to share all of my insights into what I have learned throughout the last 8 years. No matter how many difficulties you encounter, know that I also encountered some of the same things. You are not alone, and you are not an incapable parent. You can be great, as long as you embrace parenthood to its fullest potential.

The Benefits of Being Informed

- You Will Be Able to Deal with the Unexpected: Being a parent involves a lot of flexibility. While you can have the best parenting plan in the world, there will always be something that comes up that will challenge the way you think. Being able to think outside of the box is going to help you deal with the unexpected challenges that parenting throws your way.
- You will Get to Spend More Time with Your Baby: When you aren't burdened by

the worries of not knowing what to do during your baby's first year, you will actually get to spend more time bonding with your baby. During pregnancy, you should be doing all of the research you can about parenting and what to expect. If you are already prepared by the time your delivery date comes around, your sole focus can be creating that irreplaceable bond with your child.

- You will Learn the Milestones: During each month, your baby is going to hit various milestones. These include eating solid foods, teething, walking, and potentially even talking. As mentioned, even if your baby isn't at a particular milestone at the given time that the average child experiences it, you will still have an idea of what is to come. This means that there is always something to look forward to!

- You Can Learn Coping Techniques: There will be times of frustration and stress –

that's a given. You are only human, and just as your baby will, you will also feel like throwing the occasional temper tantrum. What matters is how you choose to deal with them. As a parent, you aren't going to have a lot of time to sit down and decompress. Being alone with your own thoughts for even 10 minutes can often be a challenge, so you must learn how to find solutions for your mistakes, pay attention to things that can ease your stress, and learn how to keep your baby from being fussy.

- Your Daily Routine Will Transform: A lot of parents struggle with altering their daily lifestyle in order to fit the new role of caring for a newborn. By juggling a career, managing a household, and ensuring that the baby is safe and happy, a lot of changes must be made. If you are educated before the delivery, you should not have a hard time transitioning from being in the hospital with your newborn to being at home with them. Each aspect of your life is going to change a little bit, and it is possible to make this seamless if you work on it during your pregnancy. Don't stress over this part; the transition is going to happen the way it needs to.

Do You Want to Be a Great Parent?

If you want to know if your baby is developing well, how to cope with the struggles of parenthood, deciding on whether a particular vaccine or vitamin is necessary to your child, and more, then you need to continue reading this guide. For every step of the way, this guide is going to provide you with helpful and important information that is not only meant to educate you, but it is also meant to show you that you are not alone. You are not the only parent in the world who feels this way, and that is a promise. The solutions and tips you will find are meant to be used right away. As soon as you begin to implement them, you will notice that parenting is going to feel more natural.

By reading this book right now, you are securing a great future for your baby. Be proud of yourself for this because it is definitely an accomplishment! Most new parents don't give themselves enough credit in the beginning. Certain things are going to catch you off guard, but you will realize that your parental instincts will kick in right away. As soon as you have your baby in your arms, you will know what to do and how to do it. If you ever come to a point where you do not, then believe in your ability to learn how.

Much like being a great adult, being a great parent involves a lot of trial and error. No one tends to mention this about parenting, but it is true. At certain times, you will feel as though you can't do anything right. Seeing that smile on your baby's face is what will turn everything around, though. It will make all of the hard moments worth the challenge. A little giggle can be enough to turn your whole day around and remind you that you are this child's entire life right now. The smallest things that adults take for granted are what feel magical to a newborn.

Having the confidence in knowing that you are being the best parent to your child is a feeling that cannot be duplicated. In this first year of your baby's life, prepare to learn more than you will ever learn about becoming a parent. It is arguably one of the most important moments in parenting that you will ever experience. Don't forget to have fun while doing so, as well. As long as you are having fun, then you are doing something right. You'll notice that your baby is going to pick up the habit of mirroring quickly. Having a happy parent as a caregiver will healthily influence your baby.

Chapter 1: Baby's First Days

The first few days of your baby's life are going to be fascinating to both your little one and yourself. As they begin to explore how they are able to move their body and look around at their surroundings, you will begin to fall in love with them more and more each day. This is the time when you will truly get to know your baby and learn about their temperament. The first few days are important for both the baby and the parents because it is a transitional period of time. Your baby is brought into a new environment, and then your new lifestyle begins. In this chapter, we are going to go over everything that you will need to know in order to make sure that your baby is comfortable and happy.

Baby's Looks

Your baby may or may not have hair on their head when they are born. Some babies have full heads of hair, while others take several months to grow any at all. It will start to grow eventually, so don't worry about the pace that it does grow. It is not imperative to your baby's overall health. Their skin might appear wrinkled, but this is normal. The wrinkles will smooth out as your baby grows bigger. At the top of your baby's head, there will be a spot known as the "soft spot." Be careful not to put any pressure on this spot because it is incredibly fragile. Having this spot is normal for all newborns, and it will usually stay there until your baby reaches at least 7-months old. This is when their head reaches full physical development.

Another thing about your baby's head that you might notice is that it isn't perfectly rounded or symmetrical. This is also normal, and this can change as your baby's brain develops. A lot of brain growth happens during the first year of your child's life, and this can definitely change the shape of their head along the way. Be very gentle when handling your baby's neck and head because, as you know, newborns cannot support the weight of their own head in the first few months of their lives. As they get stronger, their muscles get larger and fill in the spaces that appear indented.

Any birthmarks or unique facial features that your baby has should be celebrated. These make your child special, and though they can also change over time, they are going to be identifying characteristics. Some babies are born with birthmarks while others will have porcelain skin without blemishes. No matter what your baby's skin or birthmarks look like, it won't change anything about their rate of development. You will also love them the same! Think about how incredible it is that you and your partner created this newborn and that your DNA is directly responsible for their physical appearance.

Bonding

Skin-to-skin contact is the best way to bond with your baby. Most parenting guides will tell you the same thing. This contact is exactly as it sounds — holding your baby directly onto your skin. Even if it is just an exposed shoulder, your baby having access to the touch and feel of your skin will allow them to form a stronger bond with you by allowing them to get to know you more. Plus, this contact can feel soothing for both the parent and the child. Another benefit of having this skin-to-skin contact is knowing that your baby's temperature is regular. A feverish baby is going to be hot to the touch with clammy skin. If you are in frequent physical contact with your child, you will be able to detect this sooner and potentially save your baby from having to experience illnesses.

Hold your baby all the time, not only when they are crying. This will show them that they can receive this type of physical love from you at any time, not only while they are in distress. Fussy babies tend to cry more because they are led to believe that they can only receive this type of affection when something is wrong. By showing your baby that you are going to hold them and give them physical affection frequently, they will get used to growing up this way. Instead of fighting for your love, they will realize that you are giving it to them willingly. This creates a great sense of security for your little one.

Weighing and Measuring

Immediately after your baby is born, the hospital is going to provide you with their weight and measurements. A lot of parents like to include this information on the birth announcement. While it is not necessary to do so, there is not much else that you need this information for other than to satisfy your own curiosity. Don't become too involved in believing that your baby is going to become sick or unhealthy because they are smaller or larger than the average newborn. Babies come in all shapes and sizes.

Also, genetic factors play a large role in the size of the baby that you give birth to.

During your baby's first check-up, they will be weighed and measured again. The measurements that were taken after delivery can be compared to these updated measurements in order to chart their growth. The doctor will give you an accurate account of how well your baby is developing and growing. If you have any questions or concerns about your baby's size, or if you believe that your baby's size is preventing them from getting proper nutrition, this would be the time to bring these questions up with your doctor. Try not to do too much detective work on your own because this could end up scaring you into thinking something is wrong with your baby when everything is actually just fine.

Vitamin K

Vitamin K is super important for your newborn because it helps blood clot quickly. If your baby gets a small scratch, their fragile skin will likely bleed a lot. Blood that clots quickly is important because it will prevent infections. After your baby is born, at your request, they can be given a vitamin K injection at the hospital. Most of the time, this service will be free if you have health insurance and give birth at a public hospital. No matter how healthy the mother was during pregnancy, it is just not possible for the baby to have received enough vitamin K in the womb. This is why a lot of mothers opt for vitamin K injection after birth.

Your baby is not required to have vitamin K, but it is something that you should consider for their well-being. The ability to locate and stop the bleeding right away is useful for any parent, but especially a parent with a newborn since they are so tiny. If you do decide to get your baby the vitamin K injection, they will usually receive one dose after birth, one 3-5 days later, and one four weeks later.

With decades of testing, there have been no links to any side effects that have been seen in babies who have been given the vitamin K injection. While it is essential for all newborns, premature babies might need it in smaller doses. The decision is a big one to make, and it will likely be one of your first big decisions as a parent. If you do not opt for the injection, look out for any bleeding or bruising in the first few days of your baby being at home. If you notice this, it might mean that you need to go back to get them the vitamin K injection after all. Consult your doctor if you are still undecided.

Cord Blood Collection

There are four different possible blood types that everybody is born with — A, B, AB, and O. Of these blood types, there can also be positive and negative variations. Blood types are inherited, and they allow you to know if you are either RH positive or RH negative. This stands for your Rhesus factor, and it indicates whether you have a protein called "D antigen" on the surface of your red blood cells. Your RH factor doesn't impact your body during your daily life, but when you are delivering a baby, it matters a lot.

What this means for your baby is that they are either going to be RH positive or RH negative, as well. If the two of you have different RH factors, you might face some complications if your baby's blood enters your bloodstream during birth. This can happen through the umbilical cord. Any remaining blood that is in the cord as your child is born can accidentally be transferred into your body (known as a "cord blood collection"). If you are RH negative, your body will begin to produce antibodies to ward off the positive cells; this can lead you to feel unwell. RH positive women typically don't experience any complications.

While it is nothing to be majorly concerned about, there are injections that can be given to the mother at the 28th and 34th weeks of her pregnancy to help prevent this potential complication. It will usually be offered to an RH negative mother with an RH positive partner. It is predicted that two partners who have opposing RH factors are going to likely conceive a baby that has a different RH factor than the mother. While this isn't always the case, receiving the injection is simply a precautionary measure. The injection is safe for both the mother and the baby, but know that it is not mandatory. You can ask your doctor if they recommend that you get it.

Feeding

The idea of feeding your baby might seem simple, but it has been the experience of many new mothers around the world that the baby just won't latch on or create a proper feeding schedule. Don't worry, you are going to get the hang of this all. Since you are still going to be in a transitional stage within the first few days of bringing your baby home, try not to let this stress you out. Both of you are going to be bonding and learning about one another. Through trial and error, you will learn what it takes to get your baby to latch on. You will also be able to identify what the different cries mean – not all of them are an indication of hunger.

Newborns must be fed every 2-3 hours, and it is up to you to regulate this because you will be the source of their nutrition. Know that it is normal in the beginning to need to feed your baby a little bit more frequently in order to soothe them. Once they realize that feeding, much like affection, will be given regularly, then they will start to settle into some type of a comfortable schedule. If your baby doesn't want to eat at first, don't worry because they will let you know when they are truly hungry. As they learn that you have their food, they will develop different ways to let you know.

Sleeping

Say goodbye to your sleep schedule as you know it. Every parent undergoes the big change of completely uprooting their sleep schedule in order to accommodate their child. In the first few days, you can expect sleep to be sporadic for both the parents and the newborn. Some people say that their baby sleeps great and often after the first few days of giving birth, while others will tell you the complete opposite. As you know, there are no standards for comparison. Your baby is either going to be a great sleeper, or they aren't.

Try to put your baby down for a nap after each feeding. This will provide them will a full stomach which can be soothing and encouraging. If you try to put a baby down who hasn't eaten in a few hours, you likely won't have much luck. Your baby either won't fall asleep or won't stay asleep long. Through many experiments, you will learn which toys, songs, and methods your baby will fall asleep best to.

If you need a nap, take a nap when your baby is asleep. This is part of parenting 101, and it can save you from being overcome by total exhaustion. The best time to rest is when you know that your baby is resting. Any other time, you are going to need to be alert and paying close attention to your baby and their needs.

Apgar Scores

Apgar scores sound intimidating but don't worry, they do not reflect on how well you delivered your baby. To figure out the scores, the baby is checked at the 1-minute mark, as well as the 5-minute mark to see if anything has changed. In order to come up with the number, the doctor will check the following on your baby: skin color, heart rate, reflexes/responsiveness, muscle tone, and breathing rate. An Apgar score is what the doctor uses to assess your newborn's health. This is what alerts the medical team as to whether or not your baby requires additional care after they are born.

The rating scale goes from 0-10, with 10 being the highest. A score of 7+ for a newborn is normal. Anything lower than this might trigger the need for extra care after they are born. If your baby scores 6 or less at the 1-minute mark, this is often taken into account and then compared to the 5-minute score before making any final decisions on additional care. By the time the second number is given, your baby should be scoring no less than 7. While it may sound complex, it is truly a simple system that medical professionals use to gauge your baby's overall health once out of the womb.

It can be scary to hear that your baby's Apgar scores are low, but know that this is simply a guide for doctors to follow in order to best know how to help your baby if they are in need of treatment. The first few minutes of a baby's life can change in the blink of an eye, so knowing how to proceed is crucial. This is why the scores are given so early. Being knowledgeable about the Apgar scoring system, you won't need to feel any confusion or concern when you hear the medical staff talking about your baby's scores immediately after you give birth. If you are curious, you can ask them about the scores and how they have or have not changed.

Senses

You might be curious as to what your baby can see, hear, feel, and taste in the first few days of their life. Their senses are in their earliest stage of development as they adjust to being outside of the womb. Since your baby has been hearing your voice for nearly a year now, they might become very responsive when they hear it in person. Your baby's strongest sense will probably be their hearing; this is normal for most newborns within the first few days of life. Their vision will be blurry, but they will be able to see things that are around 1-foot away from them. In terms of smell and taste, your baby is likely going to be experiencing the amniotic fluid and your colostrum, both have been said to taste similar.

Your newborn is going to develop their senses very quickly after this. Within a week, they will be able to see more clearly and hear even better than before. They will have tasted breast milk and your skin if you intend on breastfeeding.

They will also likely know what it feels like to put their toes and fingers in their mouth; babies can be very curious in this way! You can expect an improvement in their senses every single day. Introduce your baby to as many new sights and sounds as you can. This is the best way to help them further develop their senses. This is your chance to teach your baby something new for the very first time.

Urine and Meconium

During the first day of your newborn baby's life, it is normal for them to pass urine and meconium. Known as the black and sticky fecal matter that your baby will pass, meconium is a perfectly normal bodily function. If you aren't expecting it in the beginning, it can appear somewhat alarming to see it in your baby's diaper. Don't worry because the texture and consistency will change as your baby adjusts to the new eating schedule. The meconium will eventually turn into newborn baby poop that you are likely more familiar with, a soft and lighter-colored stool.

You can expect your newborn's poop to change a lot in the first few days, but again, this is perfectly normal. The poop is still going to be pretty soft until your baby begins to eat solid foods. On the first day, you can probably expect your newborn to only have one poop. On the second day, this will likely increase to two. The number will increase the more that your baby is breastfed (or bottle-fed). The first few poopy diapers will likely be filled with what is known as transitional stools. These can contain blood and mucus, but there is typically no need to be alarmed. These substances can still be in your baby's body from the time of delivery.

Newborn Issues

You are likely going to be very cautious within your baby's first few days of life, of course. Every little movement and action is going to be analyzed and observed. While health issues are possible for newborn babies, knowing the signs to look for will help you remain at ease. Skin conditions are a common concern for newborns. Jaundice is known as the yellowing of the skin and eyes, and it is very normal for newborns to develop. It happens due to too much bilirubin being present in the skin. It is typically not painful or too concerning, but you should contact your doctor if you notice this yellowing.

Your doctor should also be contacted if you notice any dehydration paired with fewer wet diapers. This means that your baby isn't getting enough milk in their system. Fevers are also another sign to look for. If your baby feels warmer than usual, this is typically an early sign of infection. Newborns can reach high temperatures very quickly, so make sure that you are checking your baby's temperature often. Contact your doctor right away, and make sure you are ready to bring your baby in if their fever reaches 100-degrees or higher.

Spitting up is going to happen a lot, especially after feeding. This is how your baby has to learn how to digest in the beginning. It might look like your baby is throwing up after each feeding, but this is normal in order to regulate their body and get used to the amount of food they are receiving. This will happen less and less as your baby gets older and gets used to eating. Know that throwing up happens with more force; spitting up can result from a simple burp that leads to a little bit of excess milk coming up with it. If you notice that your baby is actually vomiting and the coloration is dark green or other abnormal colors, a visit to the doctor might be necessary.

Test Screening

In the first few days of life, all babies are tested to ensure that they are of optimal health. This is known as test screening. These tests are meant to monitor your baby's development and to ensure that everything is on track. Test screening is required in every state, and it is performed before the baby leaves the hospital. It starts with a blood test in the first 24-48 hours of life. A second blood test is performed at your baby's first check-up to compare results when your baby is around 1-2 weeks old. If your baby is born outside of a hospital, a doula or midwife will typically collect the blood sample.

Your baby will also be tested for hearing loss and congenital heart disease. Both of these tests will be done shortly after birth. The first test involves a pair of earphones and sensors to monitor your baby's reactions. The second uses a sensor to measure how much oxygen is in your baby's blood. Low oxygen levels can be an indication of a problem.

When it comes to vaccines, the HepB vaccine is typically what a newborn baby will get if you consent to it. As your baby gets older, around 2-months old, you will have the option to provide them with a lot more vaccinations if you choose, as well as the second HepB shot. This can all be discussed with your doctor if you are unsure about what is best for your baby.

Chapter 2: Baby Essentials

Having knowledge about what your baby needs is the first step to being a great parent. The second step is having all of the proper equipment. Before your baby is born, you will likely purchase, or be gifted, many different clothing options, diapers, bottles, and more. These are all essentials for taking care of your baby, and knowing which items you would like to use during the newborn stage is important. Again, these first few weeks come with many decisions for you to make as a parent. This is why doing your research ahead of time will allow you to feel well-prepared for when your baby is actually in your arms and in need of care.

Breastfeeding vs. Bottle Feeding

A big decision to make is if you wish to breastfeed your child or go straight to bottle feeding. While there are many nutritional and developmental benefits to breastfeeding, some mothers choose not to and that is okay. No matter what your decision is, the following topics will allow you to decide what is going to work best for you and your baby.

Benefits

As mentioned, whether you breastfeed or not is a personal decision. A lot of women opt for breastfeeding because it allows the baby to receive the nutrition that is coming directly from your body that the baby is already used to receiving. It is thought to be easier to digest than formula, and your body is likely naturally going to produce the breast milk anyway. Overall, breastfeeding provides you with a healthy and convenient way to feed your child. While there are plenty of reasons why a mother cannot or will not breastfeed, you need to take into account your own child and your own health and desire to breastfeed. The choice is solely up to you to make.

OB-GYNs recommend that a newborn only consumes breast milk for the first 6 months of life. After this, solid foods can be introduced, but breastfeeding can still continue until the baby reaches 1-year old. Breast milk contains certain antibodies that are known to ward off illnesses that your baby could be exposed to. It lowers your baby's risk of developing asthma and allergies. Another benefit is that breastfed babies are typically less likely to develop ear infections, respiratory conditions, and diarrhea. Taking a look at the bigger picture, it is thought that babies who drink breast milk also end up having higher IQs as they get older.

When you are at the hospital, a nurse will assist you in getting your baby to latch for the first time. This part can be intimidating for a mother who is breastfeeding for the first time. You might be wondering what the best position for feeding is, and this can be entirely up to your comfort and your baby's responsiveness. Try different positions in order to show your baby that you are trying to feed them.

Pros and Cons

There is a lot for you to take into consideration before you fully commit to breastfeeding. While it does provide your baby with several nutrients, it can also be a lot for your body to handle. Considering your baby's health is one aspect of your decision-making process, but it is rightful that you also consider your own health. Breastfeeding can lead to painful, clogged nipples and soreness that can often be very hard to soothe. Not to mention, your breasts might leak if your milk production is heavy. There is also the opposite problem of not producing enough milk. These things all depend on your own unique biology.

If you begin to experience difficulties while breastfeeding, there are plenty of ways that you can physically help your body, while also ensuring that you are pumping enough milk and preparing as best as you possibly can for feeding times. Getting enough rest and staying healthy yourself is one of the key factors in producing a healthy amount of milk for your baby. If you are stressed out, this is going to impact your production levels. Also, consider incorporating pumping into your normal daily routine, especially if you are going back to work after having your baby. You will need to ensure that your baby has enough milk to last throughout the day. If you do not breastfeed, then you will need to measure the correct amount of formula.

No matter which one you choose, your baby is eventually going to drink from a bottle with the milk that you give them. You might find that your baby will start to naturally try to hold the bottle by themselves – this is a great sign. It is a natural instinct. Position your baby so that their head is propped up as you feed them with the bottle. Don't tilt it so much that the milk pours out quickly, but keep it tilted just enough so that there is a steady flow of milk. Your baby might grab the bottle or bite the nipple to indicate that they want more milk. As they develop, they will become more interactive during bottle-feeding.

The following are some comparative pros and cons for you to review:

Breastfeeding

Pros

- The nutrition that your baby needs
- Your body is naturally producing the milk
- A bottle won't always be necessary

Cons

- Your nipples can get sore
- Your milk production can get low
- Pumping can be painful

Bottle Feeding

Pros

- You can prepare many bottles ahead of time
- It can be easier for your baby to latch
- Bottle-fed babies are usually hungry less often

Cons

- There will be potential indigestion issues
- The formula will not have the same nutrients as breast milk
- Bowel movements might be more stinky and loose

Introducing Solids

As mentioned, solids can be introduced around 6-months old. As you begin to introduce your baby to certain foods, you can also begin the transition of weaning from being breastfed or bottle-fed. If you breastfeed, it is thought that breastfeeding for as long as you can is best for your baby. Most mothers find that they begin weaning at around 1-year old, though. This is a natural part of your baby's next chapter in life.

You'll know that your baby is ready to begin eating solids and start drinking less milk when you notice the following signs:

- The ability to support their neck and head on their own
- Can hold the food in their mouth without pushing it out
- Opens their mouth when they see food coming
- Can refuse food by turning away or closing their mouth
- Starts getting hungry earlier than usual each day

Remember, weaning doesn't happen overnight. It can be a gradual process that happens in steps. Start by replacing one feeding at a time. Instead of breast milk or formula, allow your baby to eat something solid instead. This will seamlessly allow your baby to become ready for the transition without it seeming like they are getting fed less. Listen to their cues; your baby will be letting you know when they are hungry and when they've had enough to eat. If it is possible, avoid doing anything abruptly. This can confuse your baby and potentially even lessen their appetite. It is always better to wean in steps, no matter if you are breastfeeding or bottle-feeding.

Start off with simple, single ingredient foods to introduce your baby to. Make sure that you wait at least 3-5 days in between each new food introduction so you can monitor your baby for any allergies. Iron and zinc are very important for newborns, so ensure that you are selecting food with plenty of both. Baby cereal is great for this. It is typically what mothers decide to give their infant's as the first taste of solid food. Most baby cereal is prepared by mixing 1 tablespoon of cereal with 4 tablespoons of breast milk or formula. After the introduction of baby cereal, you can try giving your baby pureed fruits and vegetables, still waiting for a few days in between each food introduction.

When your baby is around 8-10 months old, you can introduce finger foods. These include soft fruits (with no skin), vegetables, pasta, crackers, cheese, meat, and dry cereal. Make sure that there are no choking hazards by giving your baby tiny pieces of the food that you would like to introduce. Foods that melt in a baby's mouth, like crackers are also a great introduction to solids. You will find out very quickly what your baby's preferences are. A bad taste and your baby will be spitting the food out and possibly even redecorating your kitchen with it.

Clothing

While there are so many cute baby clothes available for you to purchase, what you buy does matter regarding your baby's health and comfort. Know that great baby clothes do not have to be expensive. There is nothing wrong with buying packs of onesies that are cheap or affordable. A lot of parents feel the pressure to only buy the very best clothing, but remember, your baby is going to get everything dirty! This is natural, and it is definitely going to happen. Whether it is a diaper mess or a stain from feeding, all of the clothing your baby wears will need to be washed frequently. For this reason, selecting a durable material is a smart decision.

Your baby's skin is going to be very sensitive as a newborn. Try not to opt for any synthetic fabrics. Those that are breathable are typically best, like cotton. Know that your baby won't be able to regulate their body temperature as well as you can. A cool breeze to you will feel a lot colder to them, so make sure that they are dressed weather-appropriate. Bundle up if necessary, and don't forget to layer clothing so that you can remove some; if the temperature warms up suddenly. Baby's grow extremely quickly, so don't get too carried away with the quantity of the clothing that you buy. Some items might only fit your baby for a week or two before you are already moving up a size.

Learning how to properly swaddle your baby is going to come in handy. Swaddling is the action of wrapping your baby up tightly so that they feel secure. Some clothing is actually made for this, allowing you to swaddle without the help of an additional cloth or blanket. Don't forget about bibs and burp cloths. After each feeding, your baby is going to need to burp and possibly spit-up. If you do not have anything to cover your baby's clothing, you can expect to be doing three times as much laundry as usual. Buy a lot of bibs, and make sure you have plenty of burp cloths nearby at all times. These are a few things that your baby will not grow out of quickly.

You might be wondering when would be an appropriate time to go baby clothes shopping is. A lot of women choose to do this after the 12-week mark. Much like making the pregnancy announcement, waiting until this point typically indicates that your pregnancy is going well so far. While it can be tempting to go out and buy onesies the instant you get your positive pregnancy test, it is usually better to wait until you are at least well into your first trimester, possibly into your second, before you go out and buy a wardrobe for your soon-to-be newborn. Another determining factor that matters to some parents is gender. If you decide to find out the gender of your baby, you usually have to wait until this point anyway. This can allow you to decide on what kind of clothing you wish to purchase.

The way that you wash this clothing is important. As you know, your baby's skin is going to be ultra-sensitive. You can't necessarily wash their clothing the same way you would wash your own. Harsh chemicals and scents can do a lot to irritate your baby's skin. Before you wash the clothing, have it pre-soak in hot water to kill any germs or bacteria. After the soak, do a load of laundry containing only your baby's clothing with a detergent that is unscented or labeled as safe for infants. If you decide to hand-wash the clothing, the same steps can be followed. Make sure that you properly disinfect your hands before you begin.

If you want a little bit of extra reassurance, you can run your rinse cycle twice on your washing machine before taking the clothing out to dry. This will ensure that there is absolutely no more soap or residue present on the material. Also, it is best to do your baby's laundry before you do any other household laundry. This will eliminate the chances of cross-contamination. A lot of this clothing is going to be stained, so make sure that you are properly treating these stains before you throw them into the wash. This part should happen before the pre-soak, and this means that you must examine each piece of clothing before you put it in. Do some research on which natural stain removers you can use on your newborn's clothing.

Drying clothing is also very important. If you put your baby in wet or damp clothing, not only can bacteria gather, but your baby can also catch a cold or other illness. Dry your baby's clothes in the sunlight if you can. If not, make sure that you read all of the clothing labels to see which dryer settings to use. Since the clothing is so tiny, your dryer can be very powerful, potentially even ruining or shrinking the material. Each label and article of clothing might require different instructions, so make sure that you always read them.

When the clothing is brand new, it is a good idea to wash it before you put it on your baby. Since it came directly from the store, you never know who touched it and what kind of germs might still be lingering on the fabric. If you are being super careful with your baby's laundry, yet you notice that a skin allergy is still developing, consult your doctor for how to properly clean and dress your baby. You might have to take some extra steps in order to make sure that you are not further irritating your baby's skin. Typically, a lot of skin allergies can be grown out of, but it is best to be extra careful in the first few months of your baby's life.

Diapers

Much like feeding, there is a decision that you will have to make regarding your baby's diapers – disposable or cloth. At the beginning of this section, you can take a comparative look at the pros and cons of each decision:

<u>Disposable</u>

Pros

- Throw them away when they get dirty
- There are more size options
- They tend to be more breathable

Cons

- They are harsh on the environment
- Dyes and gels can cause irritation
- The pull tabs can rip easily

<u>Cloth</u>

Pros

- They are eco-friendly
- They are gentle for sensitive skin
- Waterproof bands can keep leaks in

Cons

- Cleaning them requires more effort
- You will have to do a lot more laundry
- They can be less absorbent

A lot of mothers wonder about the cost of each option, as well. It is no secret that diapers can become pretty expensive! They are essential, and you are going to need a lot of them every single day. Keeping your baby clean and changed frequently is what will prevent rashes from developing. This will also keep them soothed and relaxed. Sitting on a wet or dirty diaper for a long period of time is distressing to a newborn. In general comparison, the typical cost for a family to use disposable diapers for two years is around $2,000-$3,000. For cloth diapers, the cost is around $800-$1,000. Remember, cloth diapers do require the additional step of you cleaning them. If you opt for a cleaning service for cloth diapers, this can cost you an additional amount of money, placing you closer to the price range of using disposable diapers.

If you are considering the environmental perspective, it is clear that cloth diapers produce less waste. You are going to be contributing less to landfills, but don't forget that you are going to be using more water and electricity to clean the cloth diapers. This can be a toss-up for some parents, making the two options seem almost equal in the end. A lot of disposable diaper companies are becoming more eco-friendly at the request of their consumers. Some disposables are now actually up to 40% biodegradable, therefore producing less waste in landfills. Much like the decision to breastfeed or bottle-feed, this is solely up to you and your own personal preference. While you know the benefits of each, it is your decision as a parent to make.

No matter which diapers you decide on, you need to make sure you have a proper changing station for your little one. This includes a changing table or pad, a diaper pail, wipes, and rash relief cream or powder. The height of your changing station does matter because if it is too low, you are going to be spending a lot of time hunched over and in pain. Your table should be anywhere from 36-43 inches above the floor, depending on what is comfortable for your height. The diaper pail should also be easily accessible so that you can quickly toss the dirty diaper without having to leave your child on the table unattended.

You will go through wipes very quickly, probably more quickly than diapers. Make sure that you buy refills in bulk. Naturally, you are also going to need easy access to them during your diaper changing duties. Anything that you are going to use while changing a diaper should be within arm's reach. This means that your diaper cream or powder should also be easily accessible. Irritation is unavoidable at times, so it is important that you have something around that you can put onto your baby to safely ease this pain. It might also be a good idea to keep a hypoallergenic moisturizer nearby because chafed skin can become an issue during the diaper-wearing age.

Bathing and Skin Care

Until your baby is actively crawling, a daily bath actually isn't necessary. At first, your newborn should only need a bath around 2-3 times per week. Start out by giving your baby a sponge bath until the umbilical cord stump has healed. This happens at around 1-4 weeks after birth. A sponge bath is exactly what it sounds like, and soap isn't even necessarily needed. In a baby bath, take a sponge and gently clean your baby with warm water. After the umbilical cord stump has healed, you can start giving your baby longer baths in the baby tub.

Your baby can get cold very quickly, so make sure that you keep track of the water temperature. While you don't want the water to be scalding, you do want to make sure that it stays around 75-80 degrees. If you find that the water is getting cold but the bath isn't quite finished, you can add more warm water to reheat the tub. Make sure that you have a soft washcloth nearby, as well as a plush towel. The great thing about baby shampoo is that it often serves a dual purpose. Most baby shampoos can also be used to wash the body, as well. This needs to be within easy reach, of course. Just like diaper changes, you wouldn't want to leave your baby alone in the tub to go grab something.

Create a bathing routine. As mentioned, you won't need to bathe your newborn every single day at first. It does help to decide on giving a morning bath or night bath, though. Some babies feel more awake after a bath, ready to play and stay alert. Others become sleepy afterward. See how your baby responds, and this will help you decide when you should be giving them a bath. If you do want a bath to be a precursor to sleep, make sure that you swaddle your baby once they are dry, and keep the room dimly lit. This will promote sleepiness. You should also make sure that your baby isn't hungry or too full before bath time. They won't be able to go straight to sleep after they bathe if they are either one of these things.

Putting your baby into the tub for the first time can be a nerve-wracking experience as a parent. Your baby might react suddenly to the water since this is a new sensation, so don't panic. Holding your baby in your arms, gently slide their feet into the water first. Allow them to become acclimated to the way that it feels. With one hand supporting your baby's bottom and the other wrapped around their torso under the arms, you can gently begin lowering them into the tub. For the first few baths, don't let them last for very long. As mentioned, your baby will get cold very quickly. Quick introductions are the best way for your baby to get used to bathing.

As they get older, they will likely begin to enjoy bath time more. This becomes a great bonding experience that you can share with your baby. Try to make baths seem fun and positive. Always guard your baby's face as you rinse out any shampoo, even if it is safe on the eyes. Getting water poured directly onto the face can be a very jarring experience, so do your best to avoid it. You can begin to incorporate bath toys as your

72

baby gets old enough to enjoy them. You might notice your baby splashing and kicking in the water. This is typically a sign that they are enjoying the bath and having fun in the tub.

Your baby can get pimples, and this is normal. They can appear on your baby's cheeks, noses, and foreheads. This tends to happen during the first few months of life, and the bumps will go away on their own. Blotchy skin is something that can also happen to your baby; it will also typically go away on its own. Your baby's skin is adjusting to being outside of the womb, so certain things will irritate it very easily in the beginning. There should be no cause for alarm unless it is causing your baby discomfort. Know that any sort of blemish or pimple will go away within a few days. Breakouts that are getting worse or lasting for more than a few days can be brought up with your doctor.

Once you begin bathing your baby, you might notice that their scalp is getting flaky. This is known as cradle cap. This is a normal buildup of cells that a lot of infants experience. It will usually go away on its own by the time your baby reaches the age of 1. In order to help their scalp, you can wash the flakes away with their shampoo, ensuring that you rinse it all very carefully. Cradle cap is nothing to be concerned about. If there seems to be an excessive amount of flaking that does not improve, you can ask your doctor for other solutions. Certain mineral oils are safe to use on your baby's head, and your doctor can recommend which one would work best.

You might notice that your baby's skin is irritated because they keep scratching themselves. Usually, infant mittens will fix this problem and protect them. If a nail trimming is in order, there are special nail clippers that are safe for infants. Their nails will be softer than your own, so be very gentle with them. Clip them when your baby is asleep if you'd like to have the most fuss-free experience. When cutting fingernails, follow the curve of the finger, ensuring that you aren't cutting too short. For toenails, they can be cut straight across.

Chapter 3: Healthcare, Vaccinations, and Childcare

Knowing what to do when your baby is in need of a check-up, a vaccination, or childcare are all very important parts of their first year of life. Wellness check-ups are going to happen frequently for your baby. They are meant to ensure that everything is going well developmentally, and during these visits, your doctor can recommend which vaccines are typically given at the age your baby is. Another important decision to make is who will watch your baby when you are not available. Unfortunately, many parents must return to work shortly after their baby has been born. This decision is so important because you need to make sure that you have a trustworthy and safe option for your baby.

How to Choose Your Baby's Healthcare Provider

Your baby's healthcare does not end after birth; this is only the beginning. At around three months prior to your due date, it is a good idea for you to start the search for a doctor that you can begin seeing regularly after you deliver. While some continue seeing the doctor that they currently have, a lot of people like to take a look at their options. There are several necessary check-ups that will be needed throughout your baby's first year of life, so having a regular doctor is very important. Get recommendations from everyone you know. Your loved ones might be able to provide you with some insight. Along with this, you can read reviews online from verified clients who have experienced visits with each doctor.

Options

You have one of two options when making your decision – pediatrician or family physician. If you chose the former, you can typically keep your child with them until they turn 21. Those who are trained in pediatrics have a special focus on treating babies and children. It is common for a baby to see a pediatrician, but it isn't mandatory. If you choose a family physician, this is going to be someone your child can see for life if they want to. They see patients of all ages, babies included. While both have the same amount of medical experience, they specialize in different practices. Parents normally start their babies off at a pediatrician, and then they switch to a family physician or regular physician once the child reaches puberty.

There really isn't a "better" option when it comes to who you decide to take your baby to. Through research and potential recommendations that you receive, you will be able to make a well-informed decision. Also, consider where your doctor is located. If you need to drive very far away to take your baby to the doctor, this can become an inconvenience. It can also become dangerous if you are dealing with an emergency. Having a doctor that is close-by will make your life a lot easier since you will be taking your baby there a lot in the first few months of their life. Consider that your health insurance provider can help you locate a doctor in your area. Most have searches that you can utilize that will allow you to provide a zip code and a radius that you are comfortable with.

Factors to Consider

Does your baby have any preexisting conditions? Some babies are born with certain illnesses or defects, and these must be treated properly. You might have to seek out specialty treatment depending on how healthy your baby is after delivery. If your baby was born healthy, without any apparent medical conditions, then you are going to have a lot of options. Think about your current schedule. Do you work? Does your significant other work? You need to select a doctor that has office hours that work for you. It wouldn't make sense to select a doctor who has limited time to see your baby. Being a parent, you will realize that getting rid of inconveniences is going to ultimately help your life become easier.

With the doctor you choose, consider if they are working at a solo practice or as a group. If your doctor works solo, this isn't necessarily a downfall, just know that securing an appointment might be harder. Doctors that are a part of a group practice will have more staff available to treat your child, so you can make appointments that are both scheduled and more urgent with ease. If you need to call your doctor, is there someone who will answer your call 24/7 or do the calls go unanswered while the office is closed? Some offices have a service that allows trained staff to remain available at all hours in case you call with questions. This can be very beneficial, as a lot of things can happen in your baby's first year that you'll likely want to discuss with a professional. Having this option is like having a bit of extra reassurance.

Comparing Providers

The easiest way to compare different providers is by reading online reviews. This is something you can do from home, and it allows you to read about real, first-hand experiences that were had by clients. Take a look at these first, and then make a note of the doctors that you would consider taking your child to. Once you have some options, give each one a call. Is the receptionist polite and helpful? This is important because if you have a bad experience from simply calling the front desk, it is likely that you aren't going to feel comfortable once you are actually at the office. A friendly staff is a big factor that can either make or break your experience, and it definitely should be taken into consideration.

Schedule consultations with each doctor that you'd like to meet. When you are able to talk to the doctor in person, you will be able to voice your questions and concerns. A good doctor is going to listen to you, free of judgment. You will have to decide if you feel comfortable at the office, so use your best instincts. Having your significant other there with you will automatically provide you with another opinion, so consider going to these consultations together. If you both like the doctor and feel that you can trust them, then they are probably going to be a good fit for you and your baby. Ask your loved ones if they have ever heard of any of the doctors that you are considering. Those in your life, especially those who have kids, will likely know about the reputations of the local doctors in your area. Getting their input again can be a helpful tool for you to utilize. Cost is yet another factor that you might want to keep in mind. Have an idea of your healthcare budget before you go in for any consultations.

Your Baby's Vaccinations

Today, many parents are on the fence about vaccinating their children. Since vaccinations are not mandatory, this puts a big weight on your shoulders about what you believe your baby needs and what your baby could do without. Vaccinations work by training your baby's immune system to recognize and combat viruses or bacteria that enter the body. When given a vaccination, a small amount of this particular bacteria is injected so your baby has the chance to learn how to fight it off. What is injected are known as antigens, and these antigens are all individually present in all viruses and bacteria. Through the injection of the antigens, your baby's body is going to recognize that they are foreign, and if all goes well, learn how to fight them by utilizing their immune system.

If you are undecided on whether or not you'd like to vaccinate your child, consider the following benefits:

- A Vaccination Can Be Life-Saving: In the US, 50,000 people die from vaccine-preventable diseases. These diseases can be very dangerous and they can spread quickly, so choosing not to vaccinate your baby can potentially be putting them at risk of a dire situation.

- They Won't Give You the Disease: A common myth is that getting a vaccine will actually give your baby the disease that it is designed to protect against. Just because you are being injected with the antigens does not mean you are actually taking on the disease, willingly. Vaccines are designed so that it is impossible to catch the disease from them because they use cells from a "killed" virus. Others contain live, but weakened, cells.

- Vaccines Can Help Those Around You: If you decide to vaccinate your child, you are providing them with protection that will also prevent them from becoming carriers. An unvaccinated baby, at risk of becoming ill, can actually spread the disease very quickly and put others at risk. It has been shown that a group of vaccinated people have fewer bouts of illness than a group of unvaccinated people. Overall, healthier immune systems can be seen.

Common Concerns

With all of the benefits provided, you might be wondering why some parents steer clear of vaccinations for their children. One of the main reasons is the additives involved. Some vaccines contain additives known as adjuvants. They are added to the vaccines because they help them work better. They are meant to create a stronger response from the immune system, and though this can sound questionable, these same adjuvants have been used successfully in vaccines since the 1930s. One of the most common adjuvants used today is aluminum.

Though not all vaccines contain these additives, the ones that do can produce harmful effects such as pain, swelling, and redness at the injection site or even a fever and body aches. This is why a lot of people believe that getting vaccinated will automatically make you sick with the illness that you are trying to prevent. Thinking about your baby's fragile immune system, it makes sense why you might question this process and the determination if it is really worth it, in the end, to get them vaccinated.

Another concern that has popped up recently has been the idea that vaccines can lead to Autism. This is a myth that has spread like wildfire among parents, but according to the CDC, this is not true. There is thought to be no link with vaccinations (additive or additive-free) and the developmental disorder that is Autism. There have been many studies done that aim to find links between vaccination ingredients and Autism, and to this day, there have been no common links found.

Vaccination Schedule

Birth: HepB

1 Month: HepB

2 Months: HepB, RV, DTaP, Hib, PCV13, and IPV

4 Months: RV, DTaP, Hib, PCV13, and IPV

6 Months: Hep, RV, DTaP, Hib, PCV13, and IPV, and Influenza (yearly)

1 Year: HepB, Hib, PCV13, IPV, Influenza (yearly), MMR, Varicella, and HepA

Side Effects

While the vaccinations themselves might be safe and beneficial to your baby, you must also consider any side effects that are presented. Your baby might feel unsettled or sleepy after getting a vaccination, but this shouldn't last very long. It is common for your baby to need extra rest after a visit to the doctor. Dealing with the injection site is also going to be something that can be painful for your baby. This can come with some redness and tenderness in the area, but you should easily be able to manage this pain for your baby. As mentioned, fever is also a side effect. This one should be closely monitored. If your baby starts to become feverish, you need to ensure that it does not get dangerously high. Contact your doctor right away if the fever doesn't break.

With everything considered, these side effects are particularly easy to manage. Once you become educated on all of the vaccines listed above, you should have enough knowledge to make an informed decision on what you believe your baby needs or does not need. Whether you opt for all, some, or none of the vaccines, this does not make you a bad parent. The fact that you are putting thought and careful research into your decision shows that you care deeply for your baby's health and strengthening the immune system.

While every single vaccination has risks involved, you will find that the benefits are typically greater than the risks. Even knowing this information, a lot of parents still opt to go vaccine-free today because they believe that their babies actually develop stronger immune systems this way. Since the body is left to deal with any bacteria or virus that it encounters naturally, they believe that their babies develop unique ways to fight them that pertain to their individualized immune systems and functions.

Choosing Your Childcare Provider

Selecting the best healthcare provider for your baby isn't the only important care decision that you will make. An equally important topic to consider is childcare. After you and your partner have returned to work, you must make the decision – who is going to look after your child? While some parents are fortunate enough to be able to remain at home, most do not have this opportunity. This brings forth a wide array of options and a choice that can seem intimidating to make. How can you trust someone to take care of your baby and be certain that they will be safe? This section explores all of your options and the benefits of each one.

Daycare

On average, you can expect to pay $975 each month if you decide to bring your baby to daycare. This can be a costly option for some parents, especially those on an already-tight budget. When you bring your baby to daycare, you can have the peace of mind knowing that you will have someone to rely on. A daycare operates like any other business, with hours of operation and certain professional procedures. Your baby will also get to socialize with other children at a daycare center, which can be an added bonus. The staff is going to be licensed and trained in dealing with the care of infants and children, so you can be sure that they will be safe while you are away at work. At no time should your baby be unsupervised.

Home Daycare

A home daycare only differs from a traditional daycare in one way – it is operated outside of a person's home instead of a facility. This can provide a more nurturing approach to childcare, as your baby will feel that they are still in a home environment. The amount of children present at home daycare is also usually smaller since licensing requires home daycares to take on fewer children per staff member. They can also be less expensive than traditional daycare. Since a home daycare can be more relaxed, you might have the option of flexible pick up and drop off times. On average, you can expect to pay around $650 each month for your child to attend a home daycare. Since they are a little bit more exclusive due to their size restrictions, it can be hard to find home daycares that have the space for your baby.

Nanny

When you hire a nanny, your baby gets to stay in the comfort of your own home. Depending on whether your nanny is live-in, or only comes when needed, your price point will vary. You will need to pay around $2,000-$3,000 for nanny care each month, which is considerably more expensive than the previous daycare options. When your baby is cared for by a nanny, they are receiving personalized attention. This is a person that your baby is going to bond with, and the bond can become very strong. The best part is, you won't have to worry about picking up or dropping off your baby. They will already be in the comfort of your home.

Relative

If you know of a relative who can take care of your baby, this can be a great option for childcare. Of course, pricing is going to vary with this option. You will need to come to an agreement with the individual to decide on what salary is fair. Most people pay their relatives minimum wage when they care for their children. Naturally, this option is rich in advantages. Your baby is likely already going to be familiar with this person, and there is going to be a personal interest in the care of your child because of this. Your relatives can be briefed on your particular requests for your child, respecting your parenting style when a lot of daycares or nannies wouldn't be able to abide by the same modifications.

Stay-at-Home Parent

If you can afford to stay at home with your baby, this is going to be a great option for childcare. A lot of parents just can't stand the thought of leaving their little one with a stranger or even a loved one, so they opt to stay at home and care for their child themselves. You need to consider, if you had a job prior to having a baby, you are not going to be earning these wages any longer. For some couples, this is manageable, but it does require a thorough overview of all the finances.

When you stay at home with your baby, you are going to be present for every single one of their milestones. A lot of parents are saddened by the fact that they miss these things when they have to put their babies in daycare or in the care of a nanny.

Preschool

Despite what you knew before about preschool, it can actually serve as a great option for childcare while your child is still in their first year of life. While a lot of preschools are designed to take children who are at least 4-years old, some accept babies. On average, a preschool is going to cost around $740 a month. What your child will get here is a structured curriculum, which none of the other childcare options offer. Teachers work at preschools who are trained in early childhood education, both reliable and reassuring to a working parent. This is a structured option that allows your child to have the earliest chance at learning. Lots of parents enjoy the fact that educational activities are the focus.

Chapter 4: Baby's Safety and Medical Emergency Concerns

Knowing how to keep your baby safe is something that you will instinctively learn as a parent. In the first year, it can feel like your baby is prone to all of the worst dangers out there. Thinking about all of the possibilities, you might send yourself into a panic considering all of these what-if situations. Knowing what signs to look for and what to do to keep your baby safe in various situations is going to help you stay one step ahead.

Home and Outdoor Safety

Nursery Safety

Your baby's nursery should be the safest space in the home. A safe haven for your baby to grow up in, the nursery can actually be a dangerous place if you aren't careful. The crib that you choose is essential to your baby's safety. An out-of-date crib might not have as many of the same safety features as a modern one, so saving up the money for a better crib is a good idea. Artwork can be very beautiful and a great way to engage your baby from the crib, but be careful where you hang it. There is always going to be a risk of the artwork falling onto your baby if you hang it right above or next to the crib.

In general, all other furniture needs to be anchored and baby-proof. Think about anything that might fall onto your baby while they reach their crawling stage. These things must be safely secured. The same can be said for the windows and blinds. You wouldn't want your baby accidentally getting access to the cord that controls the blinds, or worse, opening up the window. Make sure that both of these things are also baby-proofed. Anything that is loose on tables or surfaces needs to be big enough so that your baby will not choke on it. Babies love to put everything in their mouths, so choking hazards need to be taken very seriously.

Feeding Safety

Choking is a big problem for infants and babies due to their inability to fully master swallowing. They can choke on anything very easily, and this includes food. This happens because their physical development is trying to catch up with their ability to eat on their own. When you are feeding your baby, especially when they reach the solid food stage, you need to make sure that the pieces are cut up very small. Any fruit or vegetable skins can also become a choking hazard, so peel them when you can. Babies need extra safety when it comes to feeding because a bad case of choking can turn fatal. This is something that you must be very cautious about as a parent.

In terms of breastfeeding, there are also safety precautions to take. The ideal feeding situation is directly from your breast to your baby, but sometimes, you will have to pump milk so that you can have it on-hand for later. With any breast milk that you pump, make sure that the milk stays refrigerated for no longer than three days. Always sterilize your hands before you feed your baby or pump milk for your baby. The germs and bacteria on your hands can be ingested very easily. If you are warming a bottle of milk for your baby, always check the temperature by placing a drop on the inside of your own wrist first. Though it might not feel hot on the exterior, the internal temperature can burn your baby's mouth.

Bathroom Safety

The bathroom is likely one of the last places you would think to make baby-proof, but it is an important room in the house that your baby will soon be visiting frequently. Though you only have an infant at the moment, you need to ensure that you keep your baby away from any standing water. Not only are there drowning dangers but there are also electrocution dangers.

It is simply best to never leave any standing water, whether it be in the sink or bathtub. You should also make sure you do your best to prevent any slippery surfaces. There are bath mats available for this purpose. If your baby slips and falls, they could get injured very easily. Make sure that none of your bathroom cabinets can be easily opened. Many people keep cleaning supplies underneath their bathroom sink, and this can be fatal if your child ingests any of these chemicals. When you are giving your baby a bath, closely monitor the water temperature. While babies can get cold easily, they also feel very sensitive to heat. Ensure that the bathwater isn't too hot.

Yard Safety

The main way to baby-proof your yard is by making sure that you have a fenced-in area that is safe for your child. While your whole yard does not need to be fenced, the area in which your baby will be exploring and spending time in should be fenced. Within this area, make sure that you aren't putting your baby near any poisonous plants or small rocks that can be ingested. There should be enough space for you to set up a blanket or outdoor playpen so that your baby does not have direct contact with the ground. This is the easiest way to stay safe while being outside in the first year of life. And of course, constant supervision is always necessary. Turning your back for even a few minutes can result in an unfortunate accident.

General Safety

- Burns: Young babies are at a very high risk of getting burned. This has a lot to do with their mobility and curiosity. When you are cooking, always make sure that you keep the pot and pan handles inward to avoid an accidental grab by your baby. Any hot things should also be placed at the very middle of the table or counter and out of reach. Make sure that you plug all of your outlets, and don't let your child touch light bulbs or any other exposed lighting (Christmas tree lighting, for example).

- Falls: Your baby is going to fall a lot; this is normal in a child who is learning how to crawl, scoot, and walk. What you need to make sure is that they do not get hurt in the process. Use barriers, like indoor gates, to section off safe areas of your home for your baby to practice. Always use the straps and buckles in highchairs or other seats where your baby will be left. Make sure that you also pad any sharp corners of furniture in your home.

- Drowning: It does not take a lot of water for your baby to accidentally drown. In fact, it can happen when there is only 1 inch of water present. To avoid this, you need to make sure that you never take your eyes off your baby when there is water involved. If you have a pool, this should always remain fenced and locked. Your baby might see the water and want to go near it out of instinct, so it is better to be safe than sorry.

When to Seek Medical Attention

If you think that your baby is starting to get sick, this can be an awful feeling. While you want your baby to feel better, you might be wondering when to seek medical attention. It is normal that your baby catches an occasional cold or illness, but certain symptoms can be more dangerous than others. The following are some indications of when you should contact your doctor or make an appointment for your baby:

- Appetite Changes: If your baby refuses to eat for several meals in a row, then this is a sign that something could be wrong. Also, if your baby is eating poorly, you can take this as the same type of indication.
- Behavioral Changes: You know your baby better than anyone, so you can trust your maternal instinct. Your baby might

become hard to wake up or feel unusually tired, and this is definitely a big behavioral change to watch out for. Inconsolable crying can also be a cause for concern. Get to your doctor right away if you notice that your baby appears to be floppy or less responsive to their reflexes.

- Tender navel or penis: There are times when your baby's navel might get irritated and even bloody. The same can happen to the penis if you have a baby boy. Understandably, these are very concerning symptoms, so you will want to have them evaluated right away.

- Fever: For infants under 3-months old, fevers can often be deadly if left untreated. While it might seem extra precautionary, you need to seek medical attention right away for any fever that develops. In infants that are 3-6 months, a temperature of 102 or higher is considered dangerous. You would want to consult a doctor at that point. As your baby gets a little bit older, the case of a fever becomes less dangerous. You can contact your doctor if a fever of 102 or higher lasts for longer than 1 day. Whether or not they show any other symptoms, a fever is definitely something to pay attention to.

- Diarrhea: If your baby is having constant diarrhea, this could mean that there is something wrong with your baby's digestion. While it can be normal for babies to experience diarrhea sometimes, regular diarrhea can indicate that there is a problem.

- Vomiting: You are going to get used to your baby spitting up after feedings. This is an indication of good health and digestion, but if your baby is vomiting, then this becomes more dangerous. Vomiting is different from spitting up because it is more forceful. Projectile vomiting can be very alarming, as well. Contact your doctor if your baby cannot keep liquids down, especially if this lasts for 8+ hours.

- Dehydration: When your baby cries with fewer tears, has a fever, and is not able to urinate as much, this could mean that they are dehydrated. Keep an eye on their soft spot, as well. If it appears sunken in any way, this is also a sign of dehydration.

- Constipation: Much like diarrhea, occasional constipation is normal for infants. If you notice that your baby does not use the bathroom for a few days or appears to be struggling while using the bathroom, this can be a cause for concern.

- Colds: As mentioned, the occasional cold is normal. This is automatically more dangerous for infants since their immune systems aren't as strong as adults'. The time to contact your doctor comes when you notice that your baby's breathing is labored in any way or if they have nasal mucus that lasts for longer than a week and a half. Ear pain and a cough that lasts for longer than a week is also an indication that your baby might need medicine in order to get better.

- Rashes: A rash is normally an indication of an allergic reaction, but it can potentially mean that your baby has an infection. Get in touch with your doctor if your baby seems to have developed a rash out of nowhere, and definitely if it comes along with a fever.

- Eye Discharge: Any time that you notice your baby's eyes are leaking mucus, you will need to contact your doctor. You will be able to tell the difference between tears and mucus because it is a lot thicker. It can also make your baby's eyes red.

Of course, with any medical concern, you need to use your best judgment and common sense as a parent to determine when your baby should be taken to the doctor. There are some things that are direr and will require emergency care, such as uncontrollable bleeding, poisoning, seizures, unconsciousness, deep cuts or burns, major mouth and facial injuries, or lips that look blue or purple.

The most important thing is that you do not panic. Any of the above symptoms or situations can be enough to send a parent into a panic over their baby, and that is understandable. However, if you can keep the energy calm, then you will be doing what is best for your baby. Try to stay as calm as you can, and work quickly to get your baby the care they need.

Again, you might feel like you are being overly cautious, but it is better to be safe than sorry. Since your baby cannot talk to you yet, it can be hard to know exactly what is wrong. Even if it is something that turns out to be minor, you will be able to rest assured that you did everything you could do to make sure that your baby is okay.

Traveling with an Infant

Another situation that can be slightly stressful is the idea of traveling with an infant. While the same stressors of travel will apply, you will now have to ensure that you have everything that you need while you are away from home with your baby. These are some of the top tips to follow if you do intend on taking your baby on a trip:

1. Book the Right Seats: If you plan on traveling by plane, you need to figure out if you will be required to purchase a separate seat for your baby. Some airlines do not charge you for this, but others will require you to buy one, no matter how young they are. You need to have a proper car seat that is up to code and that can be taken on the plane. Know that not all car seats are designed for air travel, so ensure that you have the right kind. If you are planning on holding your baby, consider booking a window or an aisle seat – there are benefits to each one. The window seat can be a great distraction for your baby, while the aisle seat gives you easy access to the bathroom or space to move around if the baby gets fussy. A lot of airlines are very accommodating if you tell them that

you are traveling with an infant, so let them know ahead of time.

2. Pack Properly: Not only do you need to remember to bring all of your belongings for the trip, but you must also think ahead for your baby. You will need to bring everything necessary for feeding, toys, and comforts from home, changes of clothes, diapers and wipes, plus any car seats or strollers. Overall, you are going to be packing a lot more than you usually would, so keep that in mind when you are selecting a suitcase to take along. Also, consider that you might have to pay additional fees if you intend on checking in these additional items that you need to pack for your baby.

3. Bring Entertainment: Though your baby is still likely too young to be able to sit still long enough to watch a movie while you are traveling, you should bring along some sort of distraction or entertainment to keep your baby occupied. Babies tend

to get fussy very easily during any type of travel that requires long periods of sitting still, so make sure that you can bring some toys along to help you keep them engaged and happy.

4. Take Your Own Food: If possible, bring food that your baby is familiar with. If you are only breastfeeding, this becomes less of an issue. However, if your baby is already eating solids, then you need to prepare for the idea that the place you are traveling to might not have the kind of food that your baby is used to eating. In your checked luggage, you should be able to bring jars of baby food to keep the feeding schedule normal and familiar. Know that not all countries carry the same brands of baby foods, either. If you do intend on purchasing baby food when you arrive, especially if you are traveling to a foreign country, it doesn't hurt to bring some of your own food as a backup plan.

5. Select the Right Stroller: Much like cars, not all baby strollers offer the same features. If you are going on a short trip, a lightweight stroller is likely going to be just fine. It will also be easier to carry around with you. If your trip is longer, you might want to consider bringing a stroller that has plenty of storage space. When you have a heavy-duty stroller that fully reclines and allows you to bring food and toys along easily, you are going to have a much easier time transporting your baby.

6. Consider the Hotel You Book: Most hotels are very accommodating, but not all of them offer sleeping arrangements for infants. If you have a very young baby, putting them to bed in a regular bed isn't going to work. Call the hotel ahead of time to make sure that they will have a crib for you to use. Keep in mind that this crib likely won't come with linens, so you should pack your own just in case.

Another helpful tip is to book a corner room. At some point, your baby is probably going to cry. Being in a corner room limits the number of other guests you will disturb as you are trying to soothe your little one.

7. Get Vaccinations: Depending on where you are going, you should contact your doctor to double-check that your baby is properly vaccinated for the trip. Whether or not you regularly vaccinate your baby, it can be worth it to check on area-specific vaccinations because some countries are carriers for illnesses and diseases that can greatly impact your baby. Any foreign contact with these germs can cause a lot of problems, and a potential overseas emergency. To avoid this, getting vaccinated is the easiest way to make sure that they stay protected.

8. Consider How You Will Get Around: Once you reach your destination, you will likely need additional transportation as you

explore. Are you going to be taking taxis or ride-sharing? Will you rent your own car? This is why bringing a car seat is very important because you never know if your mode of transportation is going to have one available for your baby. A lot of parents prefer to rent their own car, if possible. This allows for a lot more freedom during the trip and a safer way to get around for your baby.

Chapter 5: First Trimester Milestones (1-3 Months)

As you watch your baby grow you will be amazed by not only their physical development but also their emotional development. So much growth happens on both levels as your child is in what is considered the "first trimester" of life. This is the period between 1-3 months of age, and it is filled with many notable milestones to look out for. In this section, you will become familiarized with what to expect and how to recognize any potential issues.

First Month

Milestones Chart

- Eyes tracking objects
- Gripping objects placed into the hand
- Noticing people and faces within range

- Making throaty noises
- Crying subsiding when held by a caregiver
- Displays of reflexes
- Lifting head during tummy time
- Moving limbs symmetrically
- Recognition of mother's breast

Developmental Milestones

Cognitive:

1. Expecting Feedings: In the beginning, your newborn is going to eat when you feed them. You are initially the one who is setting the intervals between feedings. By the time your baby reaches 1 month, you should start to notice that their inner body clock kicks in. They will begin to cry at certain times, indicating that they are hungry.

2. Distinguishing Tastes: Your baby will know the difference between the taste of the breast milk after you have eaten certain foods. For example, when you eat

something that alters the taste of the milk, your baby will react by either refusing to feed or making different faces.

3. Acknowledging Presence: If you hold an object up to your baby, they should be able to lock their eyes on it and focus on it. The same can be said for when a person stands within view.

4. Memory of Sensations: Your baby should now notice the difference between soft textures and rough textures. They will also respond to sweet smells differently than harsh smells.

Physical:

Your baby should be able to thrust their arms at their own will. Though the movement is jerky at this point, it is intentional. Maybe your baby will begin to make strong fists. This does not necessarily indicate any type of distress, but it means that your baby is exploring exactly what can be done with their hands.

You will also notice an improvement in their reach and aim. When you place an object near them, they will likely try to grab or hold onto it. A baby who is physically healthy will enjoy reaching for things that they find enticing. Your baby might start lifting their head slightly on their own, but still won't be able to fully support its weight. This is why tummy time is important because that is how to quickly build up their muscles so that they can hold their head up on their own.

Social:

Crying is going to be the main form of communication. A cry can indicate hunger, being uncomfortable, and needing affection. They will likely respond well to familiar voices, such as your own, and can express joy at hearing it. If you are too rough while picking your baby up, they will likely be startled by this movement, sensing the roughness.

When to Be Concerned

You do not have much reason to be concerned during the first three months of development, but there are a few indicators that you need to be aware of. This is going to be a time of great exploration for your baby, and not all babies experience the same things at the same time. Some examples of when to become concerned are: feeding poorly, not blinking in response to bright lighting, stiff muscles, limp muscles, not responding to sound when fully awake, and not being able to focus on an object in close proximity.

Tips to Improve Development

Give your baby plenty of tummy time. This is going to allow them to gain enough muscle to eventually hold their head up on their own. Choose a fixed time each day to have tummy time, and stick to this regular schedule. Your baby will become familiar with the activity, and it will help strengthen nearly every muscle in their body. You can do this around 3-5 times a day if you want to. Each session should last a few minutes at a time to start out with. Keeping your baby on their tummy for too long can cause them to feel strained or fatigued. In order to capture their interest, place a toy in front of them that they can fixate on. It becomes the motivation to reach and grasp for the object while simultaneously focusing on it and using their muscles to stay upright.

Select stimulating activities that will engage your baby. This means choosing games and toys that are bright and colorful, make interesting noises, and involve some interactivity. You should also set aside some time daily for this kind of stimulation. When your baby gets to practice with this kind of interaction, they become better able to develop quickly on both a cognitive and a physical level. Social interactions are also important. Allow your baby to meet all of your loved ones, and get them used to be held by others. You need to show them that there is safety, even when they are socializing with people other than yourself. Of course, you will want to make sure that each person who handles your baby is a positive influence with a caring nature.

Mental Leaps

At around 5 weeks, your baby will be maturing rapidly. Everything from their internal organs to their perception of the world around them will be evolving on a daily basis. They will now be able to see at a distance of around 20-30 centimeters, so you can expect a lot more curiosity to shine through. You might also notice that your baby can produce more tears than they were able to before. At the 8-week mark, your baby will have a better concept of the patterns going on around them. Everything appears to be a jumbled mess at first, but as the maturity continues, your baby will be able to pick up on the repetition that goes on around them. They should have a fairly regular feeding schedule and sleep schedule at this point.

When your baby is 12-weeks old, your baby's movements will start to change. This happens as their muscles get stronger and they realize that they have control over their body. Instead of robotic, jerking movements, your baby will likely be able to make more purposeful movements. They are also likely going to be playing with their vocal sounds a lot more. Don't be surprised if you hear noises that are already beginning to sound like words. Remember, what you say around your baby is how they are going to learn how to speak. What you expose them to at this age is very crucial. Getting to see the world from different physical perspectives becomes exciting to your baby during this stage. "Flying" your baby around the room at your arm's length can often result in plenty of giggles and amazement.

What to Expect During a Check-Up

At 1-month old, your baby is already due for their first check-up. At this first visit, you can expect a general examination. The doctor is going to take a look at your baby to make sure that all of their systems are functioning correctly and that they are responding to certain stimuli. Measurements will then be taken. The length, weight, and head circumference are recorded so that the doctor can view your baby's numbers on a growth chart to make sure everything is on track. The doctor will also monitor your baby's developmental milestones. Since you are going to have to speak for them, you need to tell your doctor what your baby has accomplished since the last visit (or since birth).

Your doctor is also going to ask you a series of questions about your baby's typical behavior. This is to rule out any behavioral disorders or any abnormal patterns of behavior. There is nothing to worry about here, and it is best to just be honest with the doctor. Mention anything that you find noteworthy. Next, the physical examination will take place. The doctor will check your baby's eyes, ears, nose, mouth, lungs, heart, abdomen, skin, genitalia, and hips/legs. While your baby still has a soft spot, this will also be examined on the head. You might be given the option to get your baby tested for tuberculosis, and if you are vaccinating, they will receive their second round of the HepB vaccine.

Second Month

Milestones Chart

- Can raise head 45-degrees when on tummy
- Holds head straight while in a supported seated position
- Places partial weight on elbows
- Can visually follow objects moving in a small arch
- Can search for sounds by turning head
- Recognize faces

- Cooing and gurgling
- Will smile at familiar faces
- Becomes fussy when bored
- Responds to voices with cooing

Developmental Milestones

Cognitive:

1. Paying Attention to Faces: When your little one looks at your face, you should experience periods of eye contact. This happens as your baby's vision continues to develop.

2. Location of Sound Source: Your baby's brain and hearing should be pretty coordinated by this point. They will likely be looking directly at whatever is causing a sound that has caught their attention.

3. Unique Crying Tones: When your baby is hungry, you will know it. The same can be said for when your baby needs a new diaper. These cries should now sound different.

Physical: Lifting the head and being able to hold the head up is one of the biggest physical milestones that your baby will experience this month. They will also begin to partially push up onto their elbows during tummy time, but likely won't be able to hold the position for a long time yet. Their vision and eye coordination should be improving daily as well. Your baby can now track slow-moving objects without a problem.

Social: Smiling is a significant social milestone that can be seen from your 2-month old. If they see a happy face smiling at them, they are likely to smile back. They might also respond to questions with cooing or gurgling. If any self-soothing behavior is beginning, you might notice that your baby is a thumb-sucker. This kind of behavior can keep your baby calm for short periods of time. Overall, your baby is starting to become more independent.

When to be Concerned

If your baby never smiles, an expressionless face can be something to worry about. This likely means that your baby cannot process what is going on around them. Not being able to hold their head up at all is also a warning sign. Though it is still going to be difficult for your 2-month old to hold the entire weight of their head up, they should be able to do it for short periods of time. If you notice these things, you definitely need to bring them up to your doctor.

Not bringing their hands to their mouth can also be a warning sign. While your baby does not need to do this frequently, it is normal for a baby at this age to want to explore moving their limbs more and chewing on their own hands and fingers. This might be an indication of possible developmental delays taking place.

At the doctor's office, bring up anything that you find to be abnormal about your baby's behavior. Even if it seems insignificant, you know your baby best. Bringing it up to the doctor and catching it early can often mean that the behavior can be corrected. This means that your baby might be able to catch up, developmentally. Of course, don't worry yourself over anything that you might think is abnormal. Your doctor will be able to confirm or deny these things for you.

Tips to Improve Development

Tummy time is a must, and you can place your baby on their tummy multiple times a day. Keep the sessions short, around 5 minutes each. You can do this 3-5 times a day, and by doing so, you are helping to strengthen virtually every muscle in your baby's body. It is a great way to allow your baby to exercise while also providing a fun playtime position. You can put one of your baby's favorite toys in front of them to encourage them to look up and hold themselves up.

Play games that are going to stimulate as many senses as possible. A great game to play is one where you stand across the room from your baby and make a noise until they are able to track you. This will help with their hearing, vision, ability to focus, and range of movement. Making these games a part of your daily routine will allow your baby to be learning while playing.

Don't be afraid to introduce your baby to new people. Believe it or not, their social skills have already started developing. Though it seems early, and you might want to keep your baby hidden away to yourself, you need to allow other people to hold and interact with your little one. This shows your baby how to build trust for other people, and it also shows them that they can trust you in return. When they are handled by others and then returned to you, it proves to them that they can be social while still remaining comfortable.

Mental Leaps

Your baby now has a better perception of what is going on in the world around them. Instead of one jumbled mess, your baby is beginning to understand what eating is, what sleep is, and so on. Babies are very keen on patterns, so maintaining a regular schedule is very important. Try to get your baby on a schedule of some sort as soon as you bring them home from the hospital. This will regulate them and allow them to better understand what is happening. Having the consciousness of what is actually going on around them is a great sign. You can expect your baby to experience more moments like this one as the month goes on.

This is the age when an infant is likely to discover their hands. You might find your little one looking at, or even chewing on their hands more than usual. In their brain, they are processing that this limb is an extension of their body. Each time they move their arms or legs and touch something beside them, they will be more likely to notice it. Movements that are made might appear a bit wooden. This hyper-awareness might cause them to temporarily lose control over their reflexes, but this is perfectly normal. They will return soon.

What to Expect During a Check-Up

The basics of measuring will take place, as usual. This is the time when you can discuss your baby's latest behaviors. Your doctor will be able to tell you if your baby is developmentally on track with where they should be, and you can express any concerns that you might be feeling. Check-ups are intended to make sure that your baby is healthy and happy, but they can also serve as a way to give you that peace of mind that you crave. Being a parent isn't an easy task, as there is a lot to worry about at any given time. Don't worry, though, because it will get easier.

This appointment, your baby will likely have to get a lot of shots. This can be somewhat upsetting, but know that it is for the sake of their health. If you do elect to vaccinate your child, you can expect a second HepB shot. They will also get an RV (rotavirus vaccine), DTaP (diphtheria and tetanus toxoids and acellular pertussis vaccine), Hib (Haemophilus influenza vaccine), PCV (pneumococcal vaccine), and IPV (invacinated poliovirus vaccine).

Your baby might surprise you at how well they do at the doctor's office. If they do cry during the shots, know that the pain is very quick and temporary. If your energy is nervous and upset, they are going to sense this. Try to put on a brave face for them, and know that they will be back in your arms soon for that comfort that you both crave.

Third Month

Milestones Chart

- Regularly lifts head 45-degrees during tummy time
- Pushes legs down when held against a flat surface
- Brings hands to mouth a lot
- Grasps objects nearby
- Can shake an object in the grasp

- Tracks moving objects within the field of vision
- Can be quiet or more reserved around strangers
- Back muscles getting stronger from tummy time
- Beginning to imitate some actions
- Supports body weight on arms

Developmental Milestones

Cognitive:

1. Recognizes Familiar Faces at a Distance: Your baby might express joy from seeing you across the room. They might do this by cooing or gurgling to let them know that they see you.

2. Locates Sounds: Frequent head-turning to locate a sound is considered a norm. Your baby should be very curious about different noises.

3. Will "Talk" Back: If you say something to your baby, you can expect a reply. Though

they cannot talk just yet, speech is coming just around the corner.

Physical: Head movements are going to be the biggest milestone during the third month. Your baby will be lifting their head more and supporting it for longer periods of time. They will be able to track objects at 180-degrees, and they should be super interested in what is going on around them. If your baby pushes their legs down a lot, this is a sign they want to stand. After standing, walking is going to come quickly! It can be very exciting to notice this.

Social: Your baby is going to be laughing a lot more, and it will be so nice to hear. It is a sign that something is amusing or pleasant to your little one. You can also expect a lot more smiling, especially at familiar faces. Your baby should regularly smile at those they interact with on a daily basis. They might become interested in other infants if given the chance to socialize with children around the same age.

When to Be Concerned

If your baby is unusually quiet, you might think that this is a great sign at first. A soothed baby will remain quiet and calm, but it won't take long for something to trigger a verbal response. When your baby seems as though they cannot gurgle or make any type of noise, then this can be an indication that something isn't right. While it can be a very slight developmental delay, it is a good thing to let your doctor know about this right away. An average 3-month old is going to be very noisy during their most active hours. They should also be expressing their delight by using their voice.

Head control is also something that you need to pay attention to. A 3-month old should have no problem with head control and preventing the head from wobbling or flopping forward. It is definitely an indication of some kind of developmental delay when your baby cannot keep their head up on their own, even for a few seconds at a time. In the meantime, make sure that you are always properly giving them support and then bring the issue up to your doctor. The same can be said if your baby is unable to hold an object. While they might drop it eventually, a 3-month old's grip should be fairly strong by now. When your baby plays, they should be holding onto their toys, maybe even bringing them to their mouth or throwing them around in delight.

Tips to Improve Development

You can help your baby by interacting with them all the time. No matter what you are doing, even if it does not directly involve your little one, practice narrating everything. When you explain things to your baby, this is going to pique their interest. Though they might not be able to understand all the concepts just yet, they are still going to be absorbing this information until it makes sense. Have regular conversations, and allow your baby the time to respond. You will find that they probably get excited when you reply back to them again.

Playing games that allow your baby to track objects will help to build this skill. For example, playing with toy cars that can move around will allow your baby to find something interesting, and this will then cause them to try to track the object. Don't go too fast, or this might seem overwhelming. You can play with moving toys with your little one every day and see how well they respond to them. Using sounds to get your baby's attention is also a great way to play.

Don't forget that tummy time is, by far, the best way to help your baby develop. Having enough tummy time each day will get your baby to the most advanced stage of development possible. This muscle-building activity is very fun for babies, and you can make it different each time by placing different toys out for your baby to reach for.

Mental Leaps

One of the biggest leaps that you will notice is how your baby begins to move. Instead of jerky or robotic movements of the limbs, the transitions will be a lot smoother. Your baby is still going to explore their range of motion by kicking or punching, but each action should feel more purposeful than it used to. Your baby will also be playing with their own vocal sounds a lot more. If you hear your baby yelling out in a shrill tone and then immediately giggling, there is no need to be alarmed. They are just testing out their vocal cords to see what they can do with them.

Play the "airplane" game with your baby. This involves flying them through the air, similar to the way that an airplane would fly, and allow them to see the room from this new point of view. Since your baby's vision and depth perception are both improving, this can be a mind-blowing experience. They will likely love this game, giggling and laughing as you make airplane sounds below them. You can fly them around different rooms of the house, changing elevation safely, as well. This is only one example of how you can mentally stimulate your little one. There are plenty of other games that you can play that will allow for the same results. Experiment and see which ones get the best reactions.

What to Expect During a Check-Up

There is actually no check-up scheduled for a 3-month old. The next time your baby will be seen by the doctor will be during their 4-month check-up. There is no need to worry because your baby is up-to-date on all of their vaccines and, as long as everything is going well developmentally, there should be no reason for you to take them to the doctor. Enjoy this month by letting your baby grow and explore as much as possible. Introduce them to new things, people, and environments. The more that you allow your baby to see, the more that they will have the chance to learn.

Of course, if you sense that something isn't right, you can call your doctor or make an appointment to take your child in. Use your best instincts to guide you through this month. This is kind of a test to the parents in terms of being able to read the signs that your baby is giving you. As long as you are paying attention and aware of what could be dangerous, then you should have no problems during this month.

This break from the doctor will give you a chance to think ahead about the next month's appointment. Are there any tests that you'd like your doctor to run on your baby? Do you want your baby to receive any particular vaccinations? Sometimes, this space between appointments gives you a great period of time to get grounded and confident in your parenting abilities.

Chapter 6: Second Trimester Milestones (4-6 Months)

You are now a parent to a baby who has reached the second trimester of their first year of life! Your little one probably has a big personality with plenty of cute traits that you are very proud of. Though you might be getting more sleep than when your child was a newborn, they still have a way of keeping you exhausted throughout the day. From tummy time to trying solid foods, this part of your baby's life is one that is going to be very memorable. A lot of milestones will be reached, and a lot of new information will be learned. Your baby is becoming a person that is an individual, and as a parent, that is one of the best feelings of accomplishment that you can imagine.

Fourth Month

Milestones Chart

- Responds to basic sounds and words
- Can support the body with arms during tummy time
- Smiles and laughs while looking at faces
- Can track nearby objects
- Can sit with support
- Makes basic movements during tummy time
- Can hold toys with both hands
- Cries differently when feeling certain emotions
- Can push legs downward when standing with support
- Watches new objects and people with curiosity

Developmental Milestones

Cognitive:

1. Understands Basic Cause and Effect: Your baby should now know that, when placed to your breast, this means it is feeding time. They should open their mouth in response.

2. Improved Memory: Your baby can now develop favorite toys, sounds, and colors. Their memory is improving daily, which gives them the ability to remember more things.

3. Purposeful Crying: A 4-month old can cry to tell you when they are hungry, fussy, sad, in need of a diaper change, or just uncomfortable. These cries will sound different.

Physical: Because of your baby's increased neck, shoulder, and back strength, they should be able to sit up straight when given assistance. Whether they are seated in a special chair or with the help of your hands, this should be fairly easy now. Their babble will also start to sound more purposeful, full of rhythmic sounds. You'll notice that they really take to words that start with the letters M, D, and B.

Social: They say imitation is the sincerest form of flattery, and this is especially true with a curious 4-month old. Your little one will now be imitating your gestures and sounds, perhaps even your facial expressions. They will also begin to display favoritism. This can apply to objects, toys, and people in their life. Though, this doesn't mean that they will ignore strangers. In fact, they might stare because they are curious. Your baby might try to get their attention to gauge their level of interest in interaction.

When to Be Concerned

If your baby displays absolutely no variety in facial expressions, this doesn't necessarily mean you have a little grumpy baby. It could mean that they actually are not able to make any facial expressions which are, of course, a sign of concern. Your baby should at least be regularly smiling, even if they have not yet mastered the other facial expressions that they can make. A lack of eye coordination is also a cause for concern at this stage in life. Your baby should be tracking objects with ease, especially if they are directly in front of them. If your baby isn't doing this, then there might be a developmental delay to blame.

The strength of your baby's neck and head should be closely monitored at all times. An average 4-month old will be regularly lifting and turning their head around. If your baby cannot do this and the head appears to be wobbly or floppy, then a doctor's input is definitely going to be necessary. Their limbs should also be fairly flexible at this point. If you notice that they are stiff to the point where your baby is unable to use them properly, then you need to ensure that they are not causing them any pain. Sometimes, this symptom can be a precursor to autism-spectrum disorders, but only your doctor will be able to confirm if that is the case.

Tips to Improve Development

When you pick up your baby's toys, tell them what each one is by name. Even if your baby isn't talking in full sentences yet, they are still able to comprehend these things that you teach them. Do the same with food and people, too. The more familiar with these things that your baby can get before actually being able to talk, the easier time they will have with expressing themselves. Try to talk to your baby as much as possible. Think about them as your little side-kick, going everywhere with you and helping you along the way. Your baby is always going to be interested in what you have to say, especially if you make your tone higher-pitched and exciting.

As your baby is sitting in your lap and practicing the act of holding themselves up, read to them from picture books. Reading is a great way to keep your baby engaged, especially if the pages are colorful or textured. Your little one should be able to feel the book and know that the pages are meant to be read. Don't let them destroy the book or rip it while you are reading. This is how they will learn their first lesson in right from wrong. It will also keep them safer, as you will find that you are constantly going to be trying to do for your baby. Teaching them the difference between right and wrong is your responsibility; they have no one else to learn from.

Mental Leaps

This next mental leap is the concept of events taking place. To a baby, an event is likely going to be on a much smaller scale than what you would consider an event to symbolize. For example, feeding time is an event for a baby. Sleeping is also an event. They will notice when these events do not take place in their usual order, so be prepared for a tantrum if you do have to change up the routine or schedule. Your baby is going to become very accustomed to their set routine, so beware if you plan on changing it. You'll have to slowly transition out of it and into the new one.

Your baby's senses are developed to a point where they will likely be responsive in more than one way. This means that a hand gesture can be accompanied by a vocal sound. Children's songs typically encourage these behaviors, so play this kind of music for your child. Sing along and perform the appropriate action. Your baby will catch on quickly and might even begin to imitate you. This is a very fun and new way to see the world, so if you notice a look of fascination on your baby's face, this is a great reaction. They are starting to learn how certain behaviors and actions interact – the meaning of cause and effect. Try to keep them engaged at all times, frequently showing them how to involve all the senses.

What to Expect During a Check-Up

Your doctor will measure your baby, standard to past check-ups. There will also be some developmental, behavioral, and psychosocial evaluations done. After all of this, there will be a physical examination. Understandably, this can be a lot on your baby, even if they are normally not very fussy at all. Make sure that you bring them in for their 4-month appointment after they get a well-rested night of sleep. Your doctor is going to need as much patience from your little one as they can get as these various characteristics are tested and observed.

There is a potential screening that you can elect to have done on your child for help with indicating anemia. It might not be applicable to your baby, but a lot of 4-month olds do receive the hematocrit or hemoglobin screening at this check-up. Your baby is also going to receive several shots again. These shots will be the next rounds of RV, DTaP, Hib, PCV, and IPV like the ones given at the 2-month appointment. This is another reason why you don't want to enter the appointment with a fussy baby. If they are fussy, they likely won't stay still enough to receive their vaccinations. Much like any other appointment that you've had, your doctor will ask you if you've noticed anything noteworthy. Even if it is something very minor, if you have an instinct to mention it, then do so.

Fifth Month

Milestones Chart

- Sits upright with support
- Rolls over from back to tummy
- Responds to sounds
- Makes a few single consonant sounds
- Tongue grows more sensitive to tastes
- Shows curiosity toward non-moving objects
- Uses basic expressions to communicate
- Flexes legs when on tummy
- Tests basic cause and effect
- Can recognize familiar faces

Developmental Milestones

Cognitive:

1. Easily Distracted: You will find your baby staring off at shiny objects a lot during this time. They will love to look at bright or shiny things, hear interesting noises, and feel new textures.

2. Language Development: Your 5-month old should now have a mini vocabulary. These simple, yet effective, mono-consonant sounds are how your baby can communicate with you other than crying. You can expect to hear things like "maa" and "gaa" coming from your baby's mouth.

3. Cause and Effect Testing: When a toy makes a noise, your baby will test this theory by either shaking it or banging it. This shows that they are putting together that the noise is coming from the toy. It's an excellent sign of healthy cognitive development.

Physical: You'll notice that your baby can fully grasp objects pretty well now. Your baby should be picking up toys and possibly even their bottle.

They will also stretch their hands out far to try and reach things that are just beyond their grasp. Since their neck muscles are stronger, they are able to hold their chest up during tummy time now. They will also be able to sit up straight with minimal support. Your 5-month old should be very strong at this point in their life, and it will show how much more they try to move and reach for things that are beyond their range of motion. If you put your baby down for tummy time, you might find that they are rolling around a lot. This is normal, and this is a great sign that they have enough strength to do so.

Social: Your baby's favorite thing is likely going to be playing with you and your partner. Familiar faces are easily recognized at this point in their life. They might start showing slight apprehension toward strangers, but this will subside, as long as you teach them that they can trust the person. Lots of emotions will be expressed at the 5-month mark, and not all of them involve crying. Your baby will display bouts of joy and laughter, fear and confusion.

They will even express boredom by losing interest in toys and switching to a new one. The more that you listen to your baby, the more expressive they will become. You need to show them that they are being heard.

When to Be Concerned

If your baby does not respond to sounds or voices, this might be an indication of hearing impairment. You can test your baby's hearing by making noises behind or beside them. See if they react to your voice from across the room. A 5-month old should be very responsive at this point in life. Another concern is poor hand control. This involves not having a strong grip. If your baby has ever grabbed your skin and pinched it hard, you know that their grip is developing very well. However, if you notice that they cannot seem to hold their toys or other objects for long periods of time, a developmental delay could be to blame.

If your baby's body is ever stiff or awkward, this could also be a cause for concern. Your baby should be more flexible than ever now, regularly reaching for objects and for you. This stiffness is especially alarming if your baby is getting plenty of tummy time, and it is advised that you visit the doctor right away. As mentioned, this is the precursor to many autism-spectrum disorders. But before you jump to any conclusions, you need to get your doctor's input. There is no need to worry about something unless your doctor tells you that something is wrong. From there, they will be able to guide you through a course of treatment.

It is abnormal if your baby does not display any affection toward you or your partner. Your baby should appear visibly happy to see you, if not audibly. If you notice that your baby does not elicit a response, then there might be a developmental delay occurring. Poor speech development is another thing to look for. If your baby isn't making mono-consonant sounds or even gurgling, then there is something wrong. A baby at this age should be at least making throaty sounds and plenty of noises. With all of these potential issues, it is very important to consult a doctor first. While the signs might alarm you, the prognosis could change very easily.

Tips to Improve Development

The very best thing you can do for your 5-month old is to allow plenty of tummy time each day. This is going to keep strengthening those necessary muscles in all parts of their body. Keep talking to your child, as well. As they develop, they are getting even closer to being able to say words and form sentences. You might see their facial expressions change as they try to imitate the words you are saying to them. By keeping up with the regular conversation, you are normalizing and encouraging speaking. Remember, what is so simple to adults is not such a simple concept to infants. You need to introduce them to these things that we have adopted as norms.

Make sure that you read to your baby frequently. Reading stimulates their mind while also encouraging the use of their imagination. While it is still early for them to be playing pretend, this phase is coming right around the corner. It all starts to happen a lot faster than you think. Brightly colored toys will also stimulate the mind and usually cause a visual expression of joy. Babies tend to favor certain colors by this age, so your little one is likely going to let you know which ones they prefer.

Try to put them in a seated position daily. This will further encourage the ability to sit on her own, without support. Much like tummy time, supported sitting helps them build up their core muscles so that they can eventually do it on their own. Continue with social development, as well. You should still be introducing your baby to as many new people as you can. This will allow them to have different experiences and develop their first few basic social skills. The most important thing is that you show your baby as many things as you can. The experiences that you give them are going to shape their outlook on life and on the world. It is a large job to take on, but it comes with many rewards. A lot of parents stress about doing enough for their children, but if you love your baby and teach them something new on a regular basis, then you are doing everything that it takes to be considered a great parent.

Mental Leaps

The mental leaps that your baby experiences this month will be relatively similar to the last. While there might not be any notable milestones reached, your baby is still learning something new every single day. When you compare your now 5-month old child to the tiny human they were when you brought them home for the first time, you will be surprised at all they have accomplished in such a short amount of time. Babies are like sponges; they crave knowledge, and they are able to absorb a lot of it. As much as you are willing to teach them, they will be willing to learn. In order to do this effectively, you need to find ways to keep them engaged and focused on what you are trying to show them.

What to Expect During a Check-Up

This is another month where a check-up isn't necessary unless you feel that your baby needs to see the doctor. The next check-up typically comes once your baby turns 6-months old. As long as you appear to have a happy and healthy baby, then you have nothing to worry about. If you feel that there are some concerning symptoms present, yet you do not want to make an appointment to see your doctor, you can always call them and see if they can provide you with some advice over the phone. Of course, in case of any emergency situations, you will need to get your baby help right away or take them to the hospital.

Sixth Month

Milestones Chart

- Can eat some fruits and vegetables
- Sitting up with no support
- Can use all fingers to hold objects
- Practices basic cause and effect
- Can recognize primary caregivers(s) face
- Makes simple vowel and consonant sounds
- Can roll in both directions
- Stretches to reach objects
- Can sleep for several consecutive hours through the night
- Has better vision and depth perception

Developmental Milestones

Cognitive:

1. More Curiosity: Your little one will be looking around a lot more and reaching for objects. You might notice some fascination in their eyes.

2. Cause and Effect: There will be more testing of cause and effect. For example, throwing toys on the ground and seeing that they can no longer reach their toys while seated.

3. Imitating Sounds: Since you are talking a lot, your baby will continue to imitate you. Some of these imitations might actually begin to sound like real words!

Physical: Your baby will now have better hand-eye coordination. They will be able to successfully and strongly grasp items that they want to reach. Their vision of color and depth perception is also greatly enhanced at this point. This is why 6-month olds are so easily distracted. One of the biggest milestones is sitting without support! Your baby should now have enough muscles to do so on their own.

Social: If you are feeling down, your baby will now be able to sense this. At around 6-months old, babies can feel empathy. The energy that you show your baby is often mirrored or an attempt to provide affection is made. It can be the sweetest thing when you have had a long day and your little one wants to keep giving you kisses. They learned from the best examples they were given!

When to Be Concerned

Though your baby might need some help sitting up every so often, especially if they accidentally fall to one side, they should definitely be very close to being able to sit up. Those with a delay in physical growth will not be able to accomplish this. A notable cause for concern is your baby's inability to hold themselves up, even despite all the tummy time given and other exercises from other supported sittings. In general, pay attention to your baby's muscle tone. Nothing on your baby's body should appear droopy or stiff. Either one of these signs can be an indication that there is something wrong.

Poor motor skills might lead you to realize that your baby has some sort of cognitive delay.

Remember, a 6-month old should be able to hold onto their toys and purposefully move them around. If you see your little one struggling to do so, or not having any interest in playing with toys, you need to mention this to your doctor right away. Social skills are another thing to pay attention to. While your baby doesn't need to love strangers, it is important that they respond to new faces in some way or another. No response is a sign that they are not registering that the person in front of them is someone new.

Tips to Improve Development

Now is your time to mix play with conversations. Structured playtime activities are great for a little one's developing brain, and they are also very fun. Be interactive when you see that your baby is curious or excited about the games that you are playing. Explain what is happening, and continue to refer to objects and people by their names. If you can get the whole family involved during playtime, this is another great way to get some social interaction in with their playtime.

164

Along with this kind of playtime, continue giving your baby plenty of tummy time. Make sure that you place several toys on the floor for your baby to interact with and reach for. They should be more interested than ever now to reach for these objects.

At this stage, your baby can try some finger foods. Make sure that you cut up any solid foods into tiny pieces to prevent choking. You will quickly learn your baby's preferences by what they seem to eat up and what they decide to spit out. It is an exciting milestone to reach and you will learn even more about your little one than you knew before. Though they are just starting out with solids, you still need to keep balance in mind. Even for a baby, a balanced diet is very important.

Mental Leaps

The biggest mental leap that your baby will experience this month is the concept of relationships. It is already well-established that you are the primary caregiver, but their ideas of other people in their lives will also be coming together. By acknowledging familiar people, you can know that your baby understands that these are loved ones. They should be able to clearly differentiate a loved one from a stranger. They will also begin to understand basic shapes. Toys that allow them to explore shapes that fit into certain holes will allow them to further explore this concept.

They will also have a better grasp of the concept of distance. This applies to both affection and playtime. If you are too far away to pick up your baby, they might become fussy until you come closer to pick them us. This is also another way that they can test out the basic concept of cause and effect. If they cannot reach a toy, they might become frustrated. You will notice this frustration by either a facial expression, grunts, or even crying. In their mind, your baby is starting to understand the way that things work and what their preferences are.

What to Expect During a Check-Up

The 6-month check-up is a milestone check-up. Along with all of the usual examinations, your baby is also due for another round of shots. These will include RV, DTaP, PCV, and potentially Hib. Your baby will also need a new dose of IPV sometime between the ages of 6-18 months. If you choose, your baby can now also receive the final dose of the HepB vaccine at some point between now and 18-months. If your appointment happens during the flu season, you can also consider getting your baby a flu shot. Though it isn't mandatory, babies can get hit with the flu very hard. It is difficult for any baby's immune system to fight off the flu, even the healthiest.

There are some screening options for you to choose from, as well. The doctor will give you the option to do a lead screening test. This will simply show you if your baby has been exposed to dangerous levels of lead at any point since birth, as this can greatly affect many factors of development. A tuberculosis test might also be offered. At this appointment, your baby might have their first tooth! In this case, your doctor will check on your baby's oral health as well.

Chapter 7: Third Trimester Milestones (7-9 Months)

You are very close to being the parent of a 1-year old. So many milestones will take place during this portion of your child's life. They are able to learn even faster than ever, and they are better able to communicate with you. Your baby should now have likes and dislikes, favorites, and things that they do not care for. Your little one is still little, but their mind is expanding to become bigger than ever.

Seventh Month

Milestones Chart

- Uses voice to express emotions
- Can understand the word "no"
- Can find partially hidden objects
- Develops a raking grasp

- Will respond to their name
- Tests out cause and effect
- Can identify tones in voices
- Has better depth perception
- Explores objects using hands and mouth

Developmental Milestones

Cognitive:

1. Finds Hidden Objects: A fun game that you can now play is hide-and-seek with toys! Hide your baby's toys under blankets and watch as their curiosity takes over

2. Exploring Objects with Hands and Mouth: This is a stage when you'll have to watch your baby extra closely. They will be putting just about anything they can into their mouth.

3. Understands Tones: When you speak sweetly to your baby, they will know that you mean this with affection. A harsher

tone will be understood as something more firm.

Physical: While your baby still likely won't be able to stand up, more weight is able to be supported by their legs. If you assist your baby in a standing position, they should feel solid and balanced. When your baby is lying down, they should be able to roll around in any direction they choose. Your little one has reached a very mobile stage! Their vision is now fully developed, meaning they can see all of the same colors as you.

Social: As mentioned, the tone is normally understood by 6 months of age. If you say the word "no" in a stern voice, your baby will understand this as a negative thing. For example, if they put something in their mouth they aren't supposed to, they should freeze in place when you tell them no. They will also be very responsive to their own name, as they should know it well by now. Group play should be exciting for your baby. This social aspect adds more fun to the games.

When to Be Concerned

Much like the months prior, not having a response to certain sounds and sights is what you primarily need to be looking for. Your baby should be a better listener than ever before, and they should be great at spotting objects and people since their color vision has fully developed. If your baby still isn't showing a response to faces, colors, objects, and such, there is a big chance that a developmental delay of some sort is occurring. Notice how your baby looks at the floor when they are seated above. Most babies at 7 months will be very curious. A lost expression or blank gaze is a concerning sign.

Everything should be going into your baby's mouth at this stage, even things that aren't supposed to at times. If your baby shows no interest or ability to do so, this is another big sign of a delay. Aside from being unable to perform the task, this is naturally going to limit the amount of nutrition that your baby is going to bc able to get. Unless you are the one who is feeding them, they will have to rely on you solely for their nourishment. A 7-month old should definitely be able to eat finger foods on their own by this point in time.

Tips to Improve Development

Do some play sit-ups. As you hold your baby in a vertical position, slowly lower them on the floor so they are flat on their back. With assistance, bring your baby back up into the vertical position. This is going to build muscle as well as curiosity. The next milestone will involve your baby being able to sit up on their own from a lying down position, and eventually, standing up. Encourage self-feeding as much as possible. Making sure that you offer your baby safe foods, place them on the feeding tray or plate in front of them and allow them to decide what they would like to eat.

Buying toys has never been more important than it is during this stage. Make sure that you are selecting age-appropriate toys that will offer stimulation and fun at the same time. Interactive toys will help your baby develop necessary motor skills. Social play is a great idea during this age. If possible, allow your baby to socialize with other children that are the same age. Keep it up with the family play sessions, as well. This is going to cut down any social anxiety your baby might still be feeling. Becoming a part of a playgroup that meets regularly can be a great way to maintain regular socialization.

Mental Leaps

Your baby should be very visually engaged at this point in their life. From the toys they play with to the images they see on TV or in picture books, they will show interest in many different activities. It might take you a long time to get your baby tired enough to sleep at night because of their undying curiosity for knowledge and discovery. Consider looking into some educational children's television. If you notice that your baby can focus on these, they are a great way to continue expanding the mind as the shows are typically interactive.

Being able to reach objects will require some effort – this should be very clear to your baby now. During tummy time, you might find them pulling on the floor or blanket below them in an effort to get closer to the toys they desire. Your baby might even be scooting or crawling by now! This is why having a fully baby-proofed home is important because your little one is going to want to take a look at everything they can. They might even want to explore these things by putting them into their mouth. When you set out toys for your baby to play with while they are on the ground, this will usually keep them away from things that are not toys.

What to Expect During a Check-Up

This is a month with no regular check-up scheduled. You should be very familiar with knowing that your baby is healthy, though. They should now be on a steady and balanced diet, paired with a regular sleep schedule. If anything changes in the routine, then you know that this can disturb your baby's health or make them feel off-balanced. Make sure that you are choosing foods that are nourishing to feed to your little one. Though it might be tempting to share sweet treats with them to get a nice reaction, it is best to stick to fruits, vegetables, and grains that will actually assist their growth and development in a more practical way.

There should be minimal fussing because you should be familiar with your baby's cues and desires. Certain patterns emerge as your baby gets older, and as a parent, you learn how to work with these things. While you can't give in to anything that your baby wants, you can learn how to soothe them and keep them happy. Sometimes, parenting involves compromise. You need to show your baby that you are the boss, but not in a mean or demanding way. It can be a hard thing to start showing disciplinary action, but your baby should understand this relationship dynamic by now.

Eighth Month

Milestones Chart

- Supports weight on both legs when in an assisted standing position
- Clearly tracks moving objects
- Can pass objects from hand to hand
- Speaks simple words
- Understands basic instructions
- Can typically say "mama" and "dada"
- Can grasp with a pincer motion
- Has separation anxiety
- Can easily get into a crawling position
- Understands the purpose of personal objects

Developmental Milestones

Cognitive:

1. Understanding Instructions: When you tell your baby to come to you, or when you tell them to put something down, it is likely they will be able to understand you. Though they might not be speaking full sentences yet, your baby has the ability to comprehend these simple requests.

2. Easily Tracks Paths: If you drop a bouncy ball, you can expect your baby to follow its path until it bounces out of view. Their vision should be sharp, and their comprehension should be at a high functioning level.

3. Pointing: Your baby might discover the ability to point at this age. If anything is exciting to your baby, you can expect pointing and some kind of verbal exclamation.

Physical: A pincer grasp is the ability to hold onto an object between the thumb and index finger. Your baby should have this mastered at 8-months old. You will likely notice them using it most during feeding times, carefully and deliberately picking up pieces of food that they want to enjoy. Whether your baby has many teeth yet or not, you will notice that a chewing motion is starting to happen when they eat. This is practice for when they move up a stage in eating.

Social: Separation anxiety is a notable milestone at this age. If you leave your baby alone or with someone else for a long period of time, they might become fussy or difficult because they miss you. While it can be necessary at times, it is normal because your baby heavily relies on you. At this point, you have taught your baby all that they know, so their trust for you is very large. This can cause an increase in shyness around new people.

When to Be Concerned

Vision is important at this age. Your baby should have great eyesight, able to spot familiar faces as well as visually exciting objects from afar. Even when things are close to your baby, if it appears that they show no reaction at all, it is likely because they cannot see clearly. Some infants do need eyeglasses, and your doctor might need to do a vision test to determine if your little one does indeed need this kind of assistance as well. The inability to track objects can often mean that something is wrong cognitively. If your baby can see but cannot track, mention this to your doctor. It can be upsetting when your baby doesn't recognize loved ones or people who are always in their lives, but this does not mean that they do not have a love for these individuals. This can be caused by a developmental delay.

When you try to place your baby on the ground vertically, they should naturally put their feet flat on the floor in a standing position. If the legs curl up in response, this is a bad sign. The same can be said if your baby tries to put weight onto their arms, but cannot hold themselves up. Any muscle stiffness is definitely an issue to be discussed at your next doctor's visit. Try to assist your baby as much as you can if you notice that they are struggling. Your doctor will be able to provide you with additional recommendations.

Tips to Improve Development

Go to new places! Take your baby to markets, stores, shops, restaurants, and more. Each new place that you go, your baby will get a new experience. They will also get the chance to see and interact with new people. Normalize the idea that you are going to see plenty of new people when you go somewhere outside of the house. Make sure that your baby isn't becoming too reliant on you for comfort during social situations. While it is perfectly normal for an infant to become shy and bury their face in a parent's chest, they should also display a sense of curiosity sometimes. A healthy balance of new places and familiar places should be fairly easy for your baby to handle and comprehend.

Try to play games with your baby that will allow them to crawl. During tummy time, put all of the toys just outside of your baby's reach. While this might lead to frustration, it can also lead to crawling! If your baby becomes too frustrated and starts to cry, you can make the game a little bit easier by bringing the objects closer. Use your best judgment. If you always move the toys when you notice frustration, your baby can mistakenly get used to this concept and might begin to think that it takes tears to get what they want. Having a good balance of making your baby work hard to get what they want and also helping them when they are in need is important.

Mental Leaps

If your baby has mastered crawling, get ready for an exciting adventure of a stage! When your baby becomes fully mobile, this will really make the comparison of holding a newborn to watching your child move around on their own seem like it happened so quickly. Let your baby explore your home safely by providing designated areas in which they can crawl around. You can section off your home by using removable gates and other means of safety in order to teach them that certain areas are off-limits. Your baby will learn to understand where they belong and where they are allowed to go. If they pick up anything dangerous, they should also respond to your basic instruction to stop or put it down.

Having a larger appetite is also another huge leap that can be seen during this age. Eager to try anything that you provide them, your baby is going to be willing to eat a lot more than they used to. Being mindful of food allergies, try to let your baby experience as many different foods as you can. It is fairly easy to keep your baby on a balanced diet when you have been doing so from the beginning, but the occasional treat isn't a bad reward. Using infant utensils, offer them to your little one and show them that they can be used to assist them with eating. While they might not get the concept at first, an introduction will prepare them for any future eating that they do.

What to Expect During a Check-Up

There is typically no scheduled check-up for an 8-month old baby, but of course, you need to use your best judgment. Using the developmental milestones chart above, you can see how well your baby is developing and if they are on the right track. Remember, not every single baby is going to follow the same path of development, but your baby should be close to the indicated developments on the chart. Otherwise, keep feeding your little one nourishing foods and make sure that they are getting enough sleep throughout the day. If you notice a little bit of extra fussiness, you might need to include some more naps in order for them to recharge. Though they are growing quickly, they are still in need of a lot of sleep.

Their muscles should be strong and stable. Your baby should also have urges to stand and might be crawling all over the house by now. Don't be surprised if they are already able to pull themselves into a standing position from inside of the crib. These are all amazing milestones that you and your little one are going to enjoy together. Remember, stiffness or lack of muscular development are the two main indicators that something might be wrong. If you notice this, then a doctor's visit might be necessary. Otherwise, enjoy this time with your baby and keep encouraging them to learn more and do more every single day. You should be able to tell when something is wrong by the way they cry or fuss, or if they cannot be consoled.

Ninth Month

Milestones Chart

- Crawls for a little while and then sits down
- Can stand with support
- Says basic words
- Can understand the word "no"
- Copies simple gestures
- Has great depth perception
- Can hold and drop objects at will
- Has favorite toys
- Moves objects from one hand to the other
- Gets nervous around new people

Developmental Milestones

Cognitive:

1. Can Copy Sounds and Gestures: Your little one should be like a parrot now. If you make a noise or a gesture toward your baby, they might be able to mirror it back to you. They might even be saying new

words on their own, which is an exciting stage to experience.

2. Understands the Word "No": The word no will now have a negative connotation behind it. Your baby should understand that when you tell them no, they need to stop what they are doing. This is their first understanding of what it means to be disciplined.

3. Loves Seeking Games: Peek-a-Boo and other hidden object games should send your baby into a frenzy of delight. These are the kind of games that should truly pique their curiosity at 9 months.

Physical: Crawling should be the biggest milestone at the 9-month mark. Your baby should easily be able to get into a crawling position and move all over the place. It might even be hard for you to keep up with them! When they need a rest, they will promptly return to a seated position without any assistance or support. Their leg muscles are also stronger than ever, allowing them into assisted standing positions. Your baby might test this by letting go of the support every so often, either resulting in a few seconds of standing up or falling back down onto their bottom. At this point, the parachute reflex has been developed. This happens when your baby's head is facing down and their arms automatically come forward to prevent injury to the head.

Social: This can be a very clingy time for the baby and the primary caregiver. They will be showing preference to you over anyone else at this stage. New people might make them nervous or even anxious. This is normal because they can also experience separation anxiety, even if they are only away from you for a few minutes at a time. You are their constant state of security and how they know to feel safe. On the same lines of favoritism, you will notice that your baby now has favorite toys and objects. They might ask for certain toys or whine until they get the desired toy. It is a very clear indication that your little one is developing their own interests and preferences. This peak is very standard at 9 months.

When to Be Concerned

Crawling and sitting are major milestones that should be achieved by this point. Even if your baby isn't doing much of it, a little desire to do so is a great sign. If you notice that your baby simply cannot do either one, then this can be concerning. Either their muscles are not strong enough, or something is cognitively wrong. This behavior can point to several medical issues, and it should be taken up with your doctor right away. The same concern can be made if your baby does not seem to put any support on their legs when placed into a standing position. Remember, if their legs just seem to curl underneath them, then this likely means that there aren't enough muscles built up to support their body weight. The grip is also very important. Your baby should be gripping onto you, their toys, and food. If they appear to have a weak grip, this can be another indication of a muscular problem. This problem might be made clear if your baby does have the urge to grip objects, but keeps dropping them accidentally.

Much like concerning issues in the past, a quiet baby at this stage is extremely abnormal. Most 9-month olds can say basic words and ask for certain objects. They will even be able to call you by name. A baby who is going through developmental issues will usually not be able to make any sounds at all, not even throaty noises or gurgling noises. If you notice that your baby can only make noise when they are crying, then this is something that needs to be mentioned to your doctor.

Your baby should be able to express delight when they see a familiar face walk into the room. Even if it is not the primary caregiver, such as yourself or your partner, your baby should still display some type of reaction toward loved ones or people who are in their lives daily. Cognitive developmental issues might be to blame if your baby seems to have no memory of people who should be considered familiar at this point. It can be an indication that there was a missed developmental milestone somewhere along the way. Your doctor will be able to officially diagnose a problem if there is one, or teach you ways in which you can help your child catch up.

Tips to Improve Development

When you set your baby up for playtime, let them play how they want to play. Whether this means banging toys together or trying to solve basic puzzles, allowing your baby to do their own exploration at this stage is a great way to promote independence. While you must always remember to keep a close eye on your little one, letting them experience their toys in a self-guided manner is going to be the best thing for them developmentally. If you are playing interactively with your baby, try to provide basic instructions. A great game you can play together is rolling a ball back and forth. Encourage your baby to roll a ball to you after you have rolled it to them. You can say something like "roll the ball to mama" to get your baby to understand what you are asking them to do.

Outdoor exploration is a must at this age! Your baby needs to know that there is a whole world that exists outside of your home. Take your baby on walks, and watch as their eyes light up at various findings in nature. As always, narrate the experience and explain what you are seeing. You can teach your baby about animals, people, plants, and trees. Spending a lot of time outdoors, if the weather permits, is a great way for your baby to gain new experiences and learn new things. This will also help to further stimulate their vision and depth perception.

As much as you probably enjoy feeding your little one, the time has come to let them take the lead. When it comes to feeding time, unless you are still breastfeeding, let your baby feed themselves. Cut up food into small pieces, and place them in front of your baby. This will teach them that they need to pick up the food and place it into their mouth if they want to eat it because you aren't always going to be there to do it for them. A lot of parents struggle to let this happen but know that it is best for the baby to learn a little bit of independence at this age. Of course, if your baby is fussy or struggling too much, you can offer a little bit of assistance. For the most part, your baby should be eating on their own though.

Mental Leaps

Your baby should know about the basic concepts of categorization. For example, they will know that animals are cats, dogs, horses, and cows, but they should now that these are all individually very different animals. The same can be said for colors and shapes. Keep encouraging your baby to play games that allow for some exploration with categorization. There are many games and toys that are designed for babies this age to sort objects or place them in the correct category. One of the best toys to further develop this skill is the kind that allows for your baby to place blocks into holes of the appropriate shape. Previously, your baby would likely just pick up the pieces and bang them together or chew on them. Now, their mind is more developed. You will be able to watch in amazement as your 9-month old is able to sort through all of the shapes by placing them in the correct spots.

As mentioned, taking your baby out into the world is very important. A lot of parents do want to take a more sheltered approach to parenting in order to keep their children safe but know when you keep your baby too sheltered, you are also preventing them from developing a healthy perception of the world. Small outings are great for your baby and great for mental stimulation. It is a big world out there, and the thought that one day your little one is going to be exploring it on their own might make you feel nervous, think about this as your chance to prepare them for what they can expect to see and experience.

Everywhere you go, take your baby along with you. This will give them the best chance of experiencing even more mental leaps. There are certain places that you might not be able to visit just yet, such as a movie theater, but most other places that you would commonly visit are going to be appropriate. If you notice that your baby appears curious about something, allow them to see it and experience it, if possible. Let them feel new textures and see different sights. The best thing that you can do as a parent at this point is to let your little one take the lead. Go where their curiosity takes you, and have fun while you do it.

What to Expect During a Check-Up

This is a milestone check-up, and you can expect the same procedures to take place in the beginning. Your baby will be weighed and measured, and they will also be given the usual exams that take place during typical doctor's appointments. There is one big development screening that will be offered to you. It is unlike the other screenings you have been offered in the past because it is meant to look at your baby's development overall instead of testing for one specific issue. It is a more formal test, and a lot of parents do opt for this in order to see if their little one is developing correctly and healthily.

The doctor will start by asking you a series of questions. These questions should revolve around your baby's growth and behavior. They might also ask you to play with your little one right there in the office to see how your baby responds to certain stimulation. Don't be nervous about this because it isn't a pass/fail test. This is simply a way for the doctor to see if your baby is where they should be on the developmental chart. Try to remain as calm and natural as possible because your nervous energy might end up making your baby nervous. You both know one another best, so stay strong for your baby. Depending on the results you get, you might have to put your baby through some additional screenings to rule out certain delays or impairments.

If your baby has yet to receive their final HepB vaccine, they will receive it at this appointment. Unlike past visits, your baby won't have to get many shots this time. The next shot they might receive is the final dose of IPV if they haven't had it already. It is likely that your baby has a mouth full of developing teeth by now, so your doctor will probably do a basic oral exam to ensure that their teeth are growing properly. Unless you request any other specific screening or vaccinations, this should be all that your baby needs to receive at this appointment. Your baby should be used to coming to the doctor by now. A little bit of anxiety is normal because they might associate getting shots with coming to the doctor, but you can calm their nerves by allowing them to bring their favorite toy along with them for the ride.

Chapter 8: Fourth Trimester Milestones (10-12 Months)

On the verge of turning 1-year old, your baby is probably going to start walking any day now. This is an exciting milestone that many parents wait on the edge of their seats for. Your little one isn't so little anymore, displaying favoritism and prioritization. You can tell that their mind is working extra hard to make sense of all that is happening around them as they try to figure out what their role is in this world. Your baby is likely going to be talking up a storm, as well. They will love to exercise their vocal cords, so be very vocal with them as well. Encourage them to use their voice as much as possible because this will prevent communication that stems from crying.

Tenth Month

Milestones Chart

- Crawls and pulls up to stand
- Understands the meanings of some words
- Can move from tummy to a sitting position
- Understands requests
- Searches for hidden objects
- Has some teeth

Developmental Milestones

Cognitive:

1. Understands Object Permanence: Your baby now understands that a hidden object continues to exist and that it can be found if searched for. This is a brand new milestone for this age.

2. Associates Meanings with Words: Simple words such as "no," "go," and "hi" will have a meaning to your baby. Instead of simply hearing sounds, your baby will

have a deeper understanding of what you are saying.

3. Understands Requests: If you ask your baby to do something or to hand you something, this is a request that a 10-month old should be able to handle. Even if your little one can't repeat the request, there is still a sense of understanding the present.

Physical: Your little one should be crawling a lot by this point. There might even be some chance that your baby is pulling themselves up into a standing position. By taking a few wobbly steps, your baby might be experimenting with the idea of walking. Their muscle development should be very strong, and they will leave no space unexplored, no matter what it takes to get there. During tummy time, your baby will have a lot of independence because of their ability to not only rollover in any direction but to actually come back up into a sitting position on their own. Their two lower central incisor teeth should likely be present by now. This makes eating different finger foods very convenient. Depending on the rate of development, your baby could have quite a few teeth by now!

Social: Waving is a new social milestone that your 10-month old is likely capable of! When someone leaves the room, your little one might wave in an adorable manner. They can also likely wave hello at this point. Keep waving to your baby when you leave and enter rooms, and they will pick up on the same habit quickly. They are going to be much more reactional to specific situations at this time. For example, if you take a toy away before they are done playing, this might elicit a response that comes with tears and a full-blown meltdown. They have a very clear intention in mind of their purpose in this world and the things that they do now. You'll notice that your baby has a wider range of reactions than before, being able to break down and comprehend certain situations with ease.

When to Be Concerned

Crawling is something that should be absolutely effortless by now. If you notice that your baby is simply not capable of it, even if they show the urge to crawl, then there is likely a problem that is preventing them from doing so. You can test your baby's ability to crawl by assisting them in a crawling position. Most 10-month olds will start crawling right away, as it is natural for the average baby. Any sign of a struggle or simply no reaction can mean that there is a developmental delay that is hindering them.

Being unable to stand is normal for a 10-month old, but with the proper support, there should be no difficulty. As you have attempted in earlier months, when you place your baby in a standing position, their leg muscles should know exactly what to do. If you notice limp muscles or an unnatural stiffness that prohibits them from standing with assistance, you need to bring this up with your doctor. Make sure you take note of anything that seems to cause your baby pain or distress when you try to place them into a standing position.

As the months go on, a silent baby becomes more worrisome. No matter what noises your baby is making, there should be some sort of indication that your baby *can* make noise at this age. If they have not begun making consonant sounds or imitating words by this point, their speech development has likely fallen behind. This can often be corrected with speech therapy, but it also might be an indication that there is a cognitive issue to blame. Without a proper diagnosis from a doctor, it is hard to know exactly what is preventing your little one from using their voice to its fullest potential.

Since your baby should now be eating a wide array of finger foods, having teeth is essential to being able to properly eat them. While your baby won't have a full set of teeth just yet, their lower central incisors should have made their debut by now. If your baby does not have them, or any teeth at all, this can be an indication of a dental problem. Dental problems can cause infants to become fussy if you try to touch their gums, possibly even giving them headaches. It can also alter their ability to graduate to eating different types of foods.

Tips to Improve Development

Give your baby space! The best thing that you can do is to widen the amount of crawling space that they have available. Clear out your living room floor and make sure that everything dangerous is placed aside. The more room your baby has to crawl, the more they are going to do it. You will notice that your baby will have more fun when there are more space and fewer obstacles in their way. Put various toys on the floor so they can crawl over to each one for a more interactive approach to crawling time. Getting a temporary indoor barrier can be a great way to keep your baby contained in a safe space.

Toys that allow your baby to walk while pushing are essential during this developmental stage. There are many car toys that allow your baby to walk behind them in order to push them forward. This is a great exercise and will continue the growth of the necessary walking muscles that are continually emerging each day. One day, you might notice that your baby is feeling particularly brave and attempting to take some steps on their own, without the support of any toys or other surfaces. Encourage this if you notice it happening.

If your baby falls down when they are attempting to walk, it is likely in your natural reaction to run over to them and pick them up. As long as there are no injuries, try to avoid doing this. It will encourage them to get back up on their own and to try again. If they get used to you rushing over each time they fall, they will learn to expect this. Walking is a milestone that signifies independence, and whether you are ready for it or not, your baby is about to be walking around the house.

Have as many meaningful conversations as you can. Your baby is a small human, and they now have the ability to understand cause and effect, empathy, and emotions. Talk to your baby as if you were talking to any other loved one. This will give them practice for their necessary social skills in the future, and that isn't as far away as it might seem. Encourage your baby to express their feelings, and allow your baby to hear and feel yours.

Mental Leaps

The biggest mental leaps you will experience this month involve the way that your baby talks to you and the way that you respond in return. Since your baby is now understanding more than ever, it is a great time to introduce new words into their vocabulary. Show them new items, new places. Their minds are ready to receive this new information, so do your best to show them new things on a regular basis. Babies are going to be curious for a very long time, so while they are in this stage, it feels great to be able to allow them to continue on a curious path.

While your baby is probably very comfortable with you and speaking to you, encourage your baby to talk to other people, too. It can be hard to overcome shyness or separation anxiety, so be present when you encourage your baby to interact with others. In a group setting, do your best to involve your baby in the conversation and show them that it is normal and a positive thing to talk to other people. They should be fairly comfortable talking to those they see on a regular basis, but they might shy away from others that they aren't as familiar with. This is normal at this age, and as long as you keep working on it, your baby will outgrow this shy phase.

The days of banging toys around just to make noise are probably over now. Your baby takes deliberate action to express particular emotions. If your baby is mad, they will let you know. If they are happy, they will also let you know.

Listen to them and be mindful of their feelings. Though they are still very young, their feelings should still be validated and acknowledged. This is a very healthy parent/child relationship to have that should continue well into the future of your parenting style. If you show them that you respect what they are feeling, they will grow accustomed to this idea. Remember, you are their teacher and everything that they will grow to know will come from the knowledge that you share with them. A lot of parents still baby talk or underestimate their baby at 10 months, but this is an impressionable little being that you have in front of you right now.

What to Expect During a Check-Up

There is no check-up scheduled for this month, typically. As always, you should be ensuring that your baby is getting enough to eat and trying new foods on a regular basis. You can introduce a little bit of what you are eating each day, as long as it is cut up into small enough pieces. When you are giving your baby a new food for the first time, always be mindful of any food allergies that you have yet to discover. Watch your baby closely for symptoms after they eat the new food, and if they seem to be having an allergic reaction, contact your doctor right away.

A few bumps and bruises are going to be common in the 10th month because of all the newfound mobility. If your baby is crawling a lot, you might need to get them some pants that provide extra support for the knees. It can be common for an infant to get bruises or sores on their knees from all of the crawlings that they will be doing. They might also experience having a sore bottom if they are trying to stand up and walk. These falls should be mainly broken by their diaper, so it is nothing to be too concerned about. Remember, babies are very accident-prone. Though they are becoming stronger every single day, you still need to be very careful when they are mobile and able to access various dangerous items around the home.

Your baby should be sleeping pretty well at this point, during nighttime hours. While they will still need an afternoon nap, you should not have to be getting up in the middle of the night as much as you used to. Self-soothing will be mastered by now, meaning that your baby can console themselves if they wake in the night and start to cry a little bit. Give them time to explore this by not immediately rushing into the nursery. Usually, a baby will comfort themselves back to sleep unless something is truly wrong. You need to use your best judgment and keep in mind that you are trying to give your baby a chance to develop their independence by not rushing to them right away. Your baby is a lot more capable than they used to be, so have trust in them.

Eleventh Month

Milestones Chart

- Stands without support
- Walks with support

- Follows basic instructions
- Manipulates objects with nimble fingers
- Addresses parents with the correct noun
- Knows the names of personal objects (toys)
- Repeats easy/small words
- Can recognize familiar faces in a group of strangers
- Displays frustration through babbling

Developmental Milestones

Cognitive:

1. Learns Names: When you say someone's name, your baby should know who you are referring to now. Familiar people will have a name associated with them.

2. Obeys Instructions: If you give your baby specific instructions, they should listen to you. This obedience shows that they respect and understand you as the parent.

3. Experiments with Language: Your baby might be coming up with a whole new

language! They will be more vocal than ever, testing out all kinds of words and sounds.

Physical: If your baby needs to change positions to reach an object, this should be done with ease. From crawling to standing to sitting, all of these positions should be possible for your little one. They will be standing more than ever now, and if you have stairs, don't be surprised if they have the desire to crawl up to see what is waiting at the top. Sectioning the house off into "safe zones" is very important during this stage of mobility.

Social: Your little one will be able to call for you by either saying "mama" or "dada" to the correct parent. They might even be able to call for their siblings and grandparents, depending on how regularly they see these familiar faces. Also, your baby will be able to spot known individuals in a crowd of other people. They will let you know by expressing excitement or delight at the discovery.

When to Be Concerned

Causes for concern are going to mirror those that you looked for last month. A lack of mobility is not a good sign, especially this far along in a baby's development. If there is a lack of standing, the desire to stand, crawling, or the desire to crawl, then you can probably gather that something is wrong. A lack of response to basic commands and a lack of vocal imitation can indicate some cognitive issues, so make sure that you are still paying attention to these things. Any problems that you will notice should be fairly obvious at this point, so do your best and use your best instinct to protect your child and contact your doctor when necessary.

Tips to Improve Development

Encourage independence as much as possible. If your baby cannot grasp a food item or cannot pick up a toy, give them a chance to experience this on their own before you jump in to help. Just like you should allow them the ability to self-soothe, they are getting older now, and it is useful to know how to do these things. Use positive reinforcement as your main tool. When your baby does something great, celebrate it! To correct negative behavior, try not to jump straight into punishment. Instead, constructively lead them to better behavior that you expect from them. This will make it clear to them what your standards and expectations are.

Continue reading new books to them, and allow them to meet even more new people. As mentioned, playgroups are a great way for your baby to socialize. These groups typically meet once or twice a week, so it is a low-commitment way to allow your baby to meet other children who are around the same age. Plus, playgroups are normally filled with many interactive games that build essential skills that are necessary for development.

Mental Leaps

Your baby should now understand processes. For example, if they want to eat something, they know that it takes a few steps to make this possible. They must pick up their spoon, put food on it, and then put it into their mouth. There should be far fewer meltdowns about these things at the 11-month mark. Your baby, for the most part, should be feeding themselves. Though you might need to step in if it gets particularly messy, babies this age do enjoy eating and using their own hands to do so.

This series of mental leaps actually requires a lot of patience from the parents. It is going to be messy, and in some cases, frustrating. It will all be worth it when your baby finally succeeds at what they have been trying to accomplish, though. You need to let them figure it out on their own unless they express true signs of distress. Sure, they will become angry because they are not able to finish simple tasks, but this is how they are going to learn.

What to Expect During a Check-Up

With no scheduled check-up this month, you can simply enjoy the month of new developments. Celebrate all of the new milestones, and always make sure that your baby knows when they are doing something great. Your baby should be fairly healthy at this point unless the occasional cold happens to find them. There should be no need to visit the doctor unless of an emergency or developmental issues that you notice while you are at home. Remember, babies can be very accident-prone, so you still must be very careful as they are mobile around the house.

Twelfth Month

Milestones Chart

- Takes a few steps alone
- Pulls up to stand
- Speaks simple words
- Can imitate actions and gestures

- Responds to simple requests
- Remembers the last location of an object
- Can use fingers to poke and point
- Has good hand-eye coordination

Developmental Milestones

Cognitive:

1. Knows Where Objects are Located: Your baby should easily be able to find objects that are typically stored in certain places. Their memory will be developed enough to allow them to remember these things.

2. Object-Noun Association: If you tell your baby to pick up a certain piece of fruit, they will be able to do this. You can test them by placing a bowl of various fruits in front of them.

3. Uses Objects Correctly: There should be no more banging of items that aren't meant to be played with. For example, your baby will know that a comb is used

for the hair now, and they might even begin combing through their own hair.

Physical: Walking should be the main milestone that you notice. Whether your child is walking with the support of your arms, the support of a toy, or all on their own, the desire to walk should be stronger than ever. They will also be able to use a wide variety of grips with nimble fingers that can point, poke, and prod. At this age, the average 1-year old should have three pairs of teeth. Even if your baby isn't quite there yet, you should be able to at least see a few pearly whites poking through their gums.

Social: If you ask your baby to pass you an object, they should be able to perform the task. The same can be said if you ask your baby to come to you or to stop doing something. Simple requests should be fairly easy to comprehend at this point. At 1-year old, your baby might start testing you. Even if they know what they are doing is wrong, they might try to push your buttons to see how you will react. Welcome to the beginning of toddlerhood!

When to Be Concerned

Nothing will have changed in what to look for as a concerning behavior by now. You can still keep an eye out on your child's muscle development, ability to stand, desire to walk, and eagerness to talk. Anything less than the above is considered abnormal for a 1-year old child. If you feel that your baby is behind in any way, you can bring this up to your doctor when you go in for your baby's 1-year check-up.

Tips to Improve Development

Let your baby play with blocks. This will stimulate them by showing them various colors and shapes. They will have to figure out which pieces fit together in order to build something. You can also give them a way to make music. A lot of parents opt for the traditional pot and wooden spoon. If you can stand the noise for a little while, let your baby go crazy on this makeshift drum. It is a fun and musical way to get your baby engaged. Another game you can play is "phone call." Pretend that you are talking on a toy phone and then pass it to your baby, this will encourage them to speak!

Mental Leaps

A series of actions will now be seen as a simple task. For example, when your baby watches you doing the dishes, they know that these dishes do not magically get cleaned; it takes a process. First, you scrub them in soapy water. Then, you dry them. Therefore, you are left with a pile of clean dishes. Let your child help you with chores as much as you can. This will get them to better understand how things work, and it will give them a sense of what it takes to make the series of events happen. When they play with toys, they should know where to locate them and how to put them back when they are finished playing. All the processes that are going on around them will make a lot more sense.

What to Expect During a Check-Up

This will be your baby's first official visit as a 1-year old! So much progress has been made. The typical procedures will be done, and then another big round of vaccinations will be given. You can expect your baby to receive the final HepB vaccine (unless they got it at the prior appointment), Hib, PCV, MMR, and HepA. Make sure that you bring plenty of toys in the room as a distraction, and potentially a special treat for afterward. These are a lot of shots to get in one visit, but your baby can handle it and will usually put on a brave face if they see mommy doing the same.

Chapter 9: You After the Delivery

Becoming a parent changes you in ways you probably wouldn't expect. While you can prepare for the sleepless nights and endless attempts to get your baby to stop throwing their toys on the floor, it also comes with a personal adjustment that you will have to make as soon as you deliver. From this point on, you are now responsible for this little being. You also need to make sure that you are taking care of yourself and managing all of the changes that you are personally dealing with. This chapter explores self-care and what you can do as a new parent during the first year.

10 Truths About the First Year of Parenthood

1. You are going to have many successes, and many failures, at the same time.

2. Your postpartum body is going to be squishy.

3. Your baby is unique and might not follow the developmental path of an average baby.

4. Childbirth is not always easy and painless; it can often be unpredictable.

5. You will need to get very comfortable with cleaning poop.

6. Accept unwanted advice, even if you truly don't want to hear it.

7. Keep stretching in order to remain flexible; you'll need to be nimble to handle your baby.

8. The most important thing for your baby is a strong support system.

9. Become uplifted by other mothers who have been in the same position.
10. Success can be found when you are willing to grow as a person.

Living on Less Sleep

One of the first things you will notice is that your sleep schedule has been dismantled as soon as you bring your newborn baby home from the hospital. Frequent feedings have you getting up out of bed multiple times throughout the night. You might be wondering – how does any sane parent have the ability to do this and still live a life of their own? Sleep management is going to be your savior here. If you are home with your baby during the day, sleep when they are sleeping. This will be a peaceful time for you to both get the rest that you rightfully deserve. If you attempt to clean up around the house or perform other chores, you might be at risk of waking the sleeping baby. Also, once that baby wakes up, they are going to be renewed with energy and ready to take on the day again, leaving you more tired than ever.

Most babies do not start sleeping through the night until they reach the age of around 3-months old. This means, for the first 3 months of their life, you are going to need to make some major adjustments to your own sleep schedule. Learn how to let go of messes and chaos. This is going to allow you to relax when you have the opportunity. A lot of new moms make the mistake of thinking that they can take care of a newborn, lose several hours of sleep each night, and also keep the house in pristine condition – this isn't realistic. Learn how to be okay with leaving clutter out for a few hours (or days) at a time. You will be able to come back to it soon.

Though it might seem ineffective at first, put your newborn on a sleep schedule. Do your best to make sure that they take regular naps, but not too close to bedtime. Before bedtime, your baby should actually be the most active. When you are ready to have them settle down, get them fed, washed, and then the sleepiness should follow. If you ever put your baby to bed hungry or dirty, you can anticipate that they will be crying again in an hour or so. You need to make them feel as comfortable as possible. It might take a little while before they catch on to their sleep schedule, but starting early is worth it. Babies need structured routines.

Being a parent is full of stress. Not only are you worrying about your baby, but you are also worrying about your household and your other loved ones. How do you manage it all? By accepting the help that you are given, you will be able to lighten your load. Trust that your partner can cook and do the dishes. When you want to meet with your friends, have them come over for lunch while simultaneously meeting the new baby. All of your plans can be modified to include your baby. This will make everything seem a lot more manageable than trying to change everything all at once.

Know that there is no such thing as a perfect parent, so get that idea out of your head. Acknowledge your efforts and know that you are doing the best you can. Parenting actually comes with its fair share of trial and error. There will be times where you will have no idea what the best decision is, but your parenting instinct should guide you toward the best option. Listen to what your gut is trying to tell you because, for the most part, it is right.

Try not to load up on caffeine or other substances that will provide you with temporary energy. While this can give you a great boost at the moment, all good things must come to an end. When you experience your energy-crash, your little one isn't going to pause to give you the chance to take a nap. Try to work with the natural flow of your new schedule. If you need to have one cup of coffee in the morning to get your day going, this is okay, as long as you don't become reliant on it throughout your entire day. Your body will adjust, and things will get easier. You can think of these first 3 months as a test because the rest is going to be smooth sailing when you are able to get your 7-9 hours of sleep again.

Recovering from Labor and Childbirth

Recovering from a C-Section

After your c-section, your abdomen will be sore, but you will likely be in great spirits. You've just delivered a baby! This is something to be proud of. Unfortunately, a sense of nausea and grogginess can also follow. C-sections patients normally need to spend 2-4 days in the hospital before heading home just for precautionary measures. You will likely be given bandages that you have to change, as well as an ointment to put on the incision so that you can take care of it from home. Regardless of the kind of delivery you had, you should be able to breastfeed your baby right away, as long as your breasts are producing milk. You should also be able to walk just fine and potentially even perform moderate exercises – listen to your body.

After two to four days of having your c-section, you should be able to safely lift your baby without tearing any stitches. To manage any pain that you have after you leave the hospital, the doctor will prescribe you with around one-week's work of pain medicine. The human body heals surprisingly quickly, as long as you do not overdo it. Know that you can have sex after giving birth via c-section, but to avoid any pain, you should wait at least 6-8 weeks. Around this same time, you should also be able to get back to your normal exercise routine. Your incision should be nothing more than a scar at this point, and you should be proud to wear it. That scar is the reason why you have a happy, healthy baby.

If you need to wash your hair and body, try to avoid baths. Being submerged in water for long periods of time can actually make your healing scab soft, and potentially cause it to come off before it is ready. Making sure that your scar scabs up is important because this is an indication that your body is doing what it can to heal the incision quickly. It might not look very pretty, but you will thank yourself for being patient at the end when you are left with a clean and non-infected scar. You might feel a sense of sadness or disappointment because you didn't deliver vaginally, but each time you feel this, take a look at your baby. You are still a mother and you still gave birth to this bundle of joy. Not everyone can have a vaginal birth experience, but you still had a birth experience that was unique to yourself and your baby.

Recovering from a Vaginal Birth

One thing that most mothers aren't prepared for is the amount that they will have to pee after giving birth vaginally. This happens because your body has been storing these fluids in a compact way to make room for your baby. After your baby has been delivered, expect your frequency to use the bathroom to increase. It is normal to pee a little bit when you cough or laugh. Your pelvic floor muscles just need to be re-strengthened, and this can be done by performing Kegels. Don't be alarmed if you start to feel cramping in your stomach after giving birth; this is an indication that your uterus is shrinking back to its normal size. These cramps can last for around 2-3 days after giving birth. Remember, your belly has stretched for a 9-month period of time, so you might look like you are still pregnant after you give birth. A healthy diet and some gentle exercise will get your stomach back to what it used to look like.

A lot of mothers worry that they won't have enough milk to feed their newborns when breastfeeding. Even after giving birth, your body and hormones are still hard at work. From the very first feeding, your body is sending signals to tell these hormones to keep producing the milk. As long as your baby is eating, then more milk is being produced. In terms of your personal comfort, you might have some soreness while seated. This also depends if you tore during the delivery or not. If you tore, you will have stitches, but they should only be painful for a couple of days until they dissolve. Expect this to be an emotional rollercoaster. You might experience joy and sadness at the same time, but know that this is all normal. You will adjust, and your baby will adjust, too. Try to get as much rest as you can in the first few weeks – you will need it.

When to Have Another Child

Having another child is a very personal decision that needs to be discussed with your partner. As you are taking care of your newborn, keep in mind that a new child is going to involve this kind of care, plus the care of your firstborn. The work is doubled, but if you want to have a big family, then you know that the sleepless nights and stress are worth it. While your partner might be ready to have another child in a year, you might feel differently because of the delivery experience you had. You need to communicate openly with one another to decide on a proper timeline for the growth of your family. Try not to think about having another child in the first 6 months of your first baby's life. Not only are you still physically healing, but you and your partner both will be very busy handling your newborn.

A lot of couples want siblings who are close in age so that they can have a great bond. Most wait at least 1 ½-2 years before conceiving again, but this all comes down to your own personal preference. Families come in all shapes and sizes. You might want to wait 1 year to have another baby, or you might want to wait for 7. Consider your finances, as well. Having babies isn't cheap! Taking a new look at your budget, post-newborn, you will get an idea of how much additional money you will need if you were to add another family member to your home. It is always better to be over-prepared than struggling when the time comes. Having a healthy savings account for emergencies is a smart and responsible thing to do as parents.

You will also need to consider your current career path. It is likely that you took maternity leave if you currently have a job, so how soon will your job allows you to take this same kind of leave again? Is this something that you can successfully accomplish without putting your career at risk or cutting the family finances in half. This is very important to consider, and as much as you want to have more babies, you must think in these realistic terms. Without a job, there will be no steady income to feed your family or take care of your babies.

Don't allow any social pressures to allow you to believe that you *need* to conceive another baby by a certain time, or that you need to conceive another baby at all. Despite all the factors involved, it is still a very personal decision that is ultimately up to you to make. Even if your partner truly wants another child, yet you do not feel physically ready, then you shouldn't be afraid to express this to them. Pregnancy and childbirth are a lot for a woman to handle, and it is natural to need quite a long break in between pregnancies so your body can regroup and get back to normal.

When you do decide to have another baby, a visit to the doctor for a check-up is a good idea. Your doctor will be able to tell you if you are in the right health and state of being in order to carry another baby. No all women are, so don't assume that your body is just naturally going to ease into pregnancy as it did the first time. Sometimes, health issues can arise after having one pregnancy, so you will want to make sure that your body can withstand another one before you end up getting pregnant.

Conclusion

You should be proud of yourself for carrying your healthy baby for all those months, working hard to deliver them, and then doing whatever it takes to provide the proper care. Being a parent is a joyous feeling, but it can also be filled with many unexpected challenges that might make you question everything you thought you knew. As long as you are able to stay calm and provide your baby with love and care, then know that you are doing your very best.

The first year of your little one's life is going to be filled with so many milestones, and this guide is going to help you every step of the way. When you feel unsure about something, you have your parental instinct and your doctor's advice to guide you toward the best decision for your child. Know that these months go by quickly, and most parents often wish they had a remote so they can press the pause button.

I love to help mothers care for their babies

because I remember so many of the joys that I experienced with my own children. This is why I compiled all the tips I learned into one easy-to-read guide. Know that you are strong enough to withstand any challenges that you face, and if you put in the effort, you are going to be able to give your child a great life. I know that things can seem uncertain at first, but you are going to get the hang of being a parent, even if you have to make adjustments to your personal life.

As you wait in anxious anticipation for your newborn baby to arrive, you should be well-prepared after reading this guide. For each month, you have a detailed outline of what you can expect, what you should be doing, and what you need to prepare for. This is what it takes to be a great parent – you should always be one step ahead of whatever is happening next.

Remember to enjoy your time with your infant because this stage does not last forever. A once-reliant little baby is soon going to develop into an independent child full of personality and their own interests. Get to know your baby and give them the same trust that they are going to give you in return. Parenting is not a one-sided job. Your baby is going to teach you just as many things as you will teach them.

It is normal to feel scared while also feeling excited to become a new parent. Both feelings are incredibly justified. Once you get into the swing of things, though, you will be able to build up your confidence and take every little smile and giggle as a sign that you are doing something right!

Having a child is one of life's great joys. As you watch your baby grow you will be amazed by not only their physical development but also their emotional development. So much growth happens on both levels as your child is in what is considered the "first-year" of life. Baby's first year is a year of wonder and firsts. First smile, first word, first solid food, first tentative steps, and many more—as your baby explores their environment and learns about the world. It's important to document your baby's milestones, not only to capture their magical moments but also for medical reasons.

Track your little one's milestones with this free **"Baby's Milestones Journal"**.

With everything the baby does for the first time, it can be difficult to decide which events are worth recording. It's also easy to miss an important baby's milestones in the chaos of new parenthood. So we've compiled a list of suggestions on how to document baby's first year and which milestones are worth documenting.

Get your **"Baby's Milestones Journal"** in PDF format by clicking the link below:

https://harleycarrparenting.com/babys-first-year-milestones/

or

Print the document and start to record your baby's important milestones and events.

This printable Baby's Milestones Journal is available in both "Baby Girl" and "Baby Boy" version.

Now, you can have your *easy to fill in* "Baby's Milestones Journal " in just one click away!

Let´s get started ...

Enjoy and Best Wishes to your parenting journey!

Harley Carr

References

10 Reasons To Get Vaccinated. (2019, November 27). Retrieved December 9, 2019, from https://www.nfid.org/immunization/10-reasons-to-get-vaccinated/

AboutKidsHealth. (2019, January 7). AboutKidsHealth. Retrieved December 9, 2019, from https://www.aboutkidshealth.ca/Article?contentid=453&language=English

Adjuvants help vaccines work better. | Vaccine Safety | CDC. (2018). Retrieved December 9, 2019, from https://www.cdc.gov/vaccinesafety/concerns/adjuvants.html

Apgar Score. (2017). Retrieved December 9, 2019, from https://www.pregnancybirthbaby.org.au/apgar-score

BabyCentre UK Staff. (2003, May 14). Recovery

after vaginal birth. Retrieved December 9, 2019, from https://www.babycentre.co.uk/a553491/recovery-after-vaginal-birth

Baby's First 24 Hours. (2018). Retrieved December 9, 2019, from https://www.pregnancybirthbaby.org.au/babys-first-24-hours

Boyd-Barrett, C. (2019, October 31). C-section healing and recovery time. Retrieved December 9, 2019, from https://www.babycenter.com/0_recovering-from-a-c-section_221.bc

Department of Health & Human Services. (2016, May 18). Immunisation – side effects. Retrieved December 9, 2019, from https://www.betterhealth.vic.gov.au/health/healthyliving/immunisation-side-effects

DiLaura, A. (2019, November 5). Creating a safe nursery: 10 mistakes to avoid. Retrieved December 9, 2019, from https://www.babycenter.com/101_creating-a-safe-nursery-10-mistakes-to-avoid_10414382.bc

Dorning, A. (2019, October 29). Childcare options: Pros, cons, and costs. Retrieved December 9, 2019, from https://www.babycenter.com/childcare-options

Easy-to-read Immunization Schedule by Vaccine for Ages Birth-6 Years | CDC. (2019, February 5). Retrieved December 9, 2019, from https://www.cdc.gov/vaccines/schedules/easy-to-read/child-easyread.html#table-child

Feeding babies and food safety. (2019). Retrieved December 10, 2019, from https://www.sahealth.sa.gov.au/wps/wcm/connect/5514158047d940a7ac79adfc651ee2b2/Feeding+babies+and+food+safety+Fact+Sheet.pdf?MOD=AJPERES

Garoo, R. (2019a, September 10). 2-Month-Old's Developmental Milestones: A Complete Guide. Retrieved December 10, 2019, from https://www.momjunction.com/articles/babys-second-month-development-guide_00101929/

Garoo, R. (2019b, September 10). 3-Month-Old

Baby Developmental Milestones - A Complete Guide. Retrieved December 10, 2019, from https://www.momjunction.com/articles/babys-third-month-a-development-guide_00102426/

Garoo, R. (2019c, September 10). 4-Month-Old Baby Developmental Milestones - A Complete Guide. Retrieved December 10, 2019, from https://www.momjunction.com/articles/babys-4th-month-a-development-guide_00104153/

Garoo, R. (2019d, September 10). 5-Month-Old Baby's Developmental Milestones - A Complete Guide. Retrieved December 10, 2019, from https://www.momjunction.com/articles/babys-5th-month-a-development-guide_00103315/

Garoo, R. (2019e, September 10). 6-Month-Old's Developmental Milestones - A Complete Guide. Retrieved December 10, 2019, from https://www.momjunction.com/articles/babys-6th-month-a-development-guide_00103340/

Garoo, R. (2019f, September 10). 7-Month-Old's Developmental Milestones: A Complete Guide. Retrieved December 10, 2019, from https://www.momjunction.com/articles/babys-7th-month-a-development-guide_00103344/

Garoo, R. (2019g, September 10). 8-Month-Old's Developmental Milestones: A Complete Guide. Retrieved December 10, 2019, from https://www.momjunction.com/articles/babys-8th-month-a-development-guide_00102825/

Garoo, R. (2019h, September 10). 9-Month-Old's Developmental Milestones - A Complete Guide. Retrieved December 10, 2019, from https://www.momjunction.com/articles/babys-9th-month-a-development-guide_00103235/

Garoo, R. (2019i, September 10). 10-Month-Old Baby Developmental Milestones - A Complete Guide. Retrieved December 10, 2019, from https://www.momjunction.com/articles/babys-10th-month-a-development-guide_00103241/

Garoo, R. (2019j, September 10). 11-Month-Old Baby's Developmental Milestones - A Complete Guide. Retrieved December 10, 2019, from https://www.momjunction.com/articles/babys-11th-month-a-development-guide_00103429/

Garoo, R. (2019k, September 10). 12-Month-Old's Developmental Milestones: A Complete Guide. Retrieved December 10, 2019, from https://www.momjunction.com/articles/babys-12th-month-a-development-guide_00101960/

Garoo, R. (2019, September 10). A Guide to One-Month-Old Babies' Milestones. Retrieved December 10, 2019, from https://www.momjunction.com/articles/babys-first-month-development-guide_00101911/

How Vaccines Work. (2019, November 22). Retrieved December 9, 2019, from https://www.publichealth.org/public-awareness/understanding-vaccines/vaccines-work/

Khan, A. (2018a, June 20). Washing Your Baby's Clothes - How to do it Rightly. Retrieved December 9, 2019, from https://parenting.firstcry.com/articles/washing-your-babys-clothes-how-to-do-it-rightly/

Mayo Clinic Staff. (2019, August 13). Sick baby? When to seek medical attention. Retrieved

December 9, 2019, from https://www.mayoclinic.org/healthy-lifestyle/infant-and-toddler-health/in-depth/healthy-baby/art-20047793

Montgomery, N. (2019, October 29). How to trim your baby's nails. Retrieved December 9, 2019, from https://www.babycenter.com/0_how-to-trim-your-babys-nails_10027.bc

Porter, L. (2018, November 6). When Should I Start Buying For Baby? Retrieved December 9, 2019, from https://www.everymum.ie/pregnancy/preparing-for-baby/when-should-i-start-buying-for-baby/

Rhesus D Negative in Pregnancy. (2018). Retrieved December 9, 2019, from https://www.pregnancybirthbaby.org.au/rhesus-d-negative-in-pregnancy

Safety at home. (2019). Retrieved December 9, 2019, from https://www.facs.nsw.gov.au/families/parentin

g/keeping-children-safe/around-the-house/chapters/at-home

Sheahan, K. (2019). Choosing a Pediatrician for Your New Baby (for Parents) - Nemours KidsHealth. Retrieved December 9, 2019, from https://kidshealth.org/en/parents/find-ped.html

Shopping Tips For Newborn Baby's Clothes. (2019). Retrieved December 9, 2019, from https://community.today.com/parentingteam/post/shopping-tips-for-newborn-babys-clothes

Solid foods: How to get your baby started. (2019, June 6). Retrieved December 9, 2019, from https://www.mayoclinic.org/healthy-lifestyle/infant-and-toddler-health/in-depth/healthy-baby/art-20046200

Taylor, R. (2008, October 28). Breastfeeding Overview. Retrieved December 9, 2019, from https://www.webmd.com/parenting/baby/nursing-basics#1

The Bump Editors. (2014, August 19). Diaper Decisions: Cloth Diapers vs. Disposable.

Retrieved December 9, 2019, from https://www.thebump.com/a/cloth-diapers-vs-disposable

Thurston, K. (2017). 10 True Things About the First Year of Parenthood. Retrieved December 9, 2019, from https://www.huffpost.com/entry/10-true-things-about-the-first-year-of-parenthood_b_4254464

Vaccines Do Not Cause Autism Concerns | Vaccine Safety | CDC. (2015). Retrieved December 9, 2019, from https://www.cdc.gov/vaccinesafety/concerns/autism.html

Vitamin K at Birth. (2018). Retrieved December 9, 2019, from https://www.pregnancybirthbaby.org.au/vitamin-k-at-birth

Weaning your child from breastfeeding - Caring for Kids. (2018). Retrieved December 9, 2019, from https://www.caringforkids.cps.ca/handouts/weaning_breastfeeding

Wears, C. (2018, February 9). Traveling With an Infant? 8 Things You Must Know Before You Go. Retrieved December 9, 2019, from https://www.flightnetwork.com/blog/traveling-with-an-infant-things-to-know-before-you-go/

WhattoExpect. (2019, January 9). Essentials for Diaper Changing Stations. Retrieved December 9, 2019, from https://www.whattoexpect.com/baby-products/diapering-potty/essentials-for-diaper-changing-stations/

What to Expect,Editors. (2019, March 30). Baby's First Bath. Retrieved December 9, 2019, from https://www.whattoexpect.com/first-year/first-bath/

Yang, S. (2014, August 19). Baby's Checkup Schedule. Retrieved December 9, 2019, from https://www.thebump.com/a/new-baby-doctor-visit-checklist

Your baby's mental leaps in the first year. (2019). Retrieved December 10, 2019, from https://www.thewonderweeks.com/babysmental-leaps-first-year/#5weeks

Made in the USA
San Bernardino, CA
14 April 2020